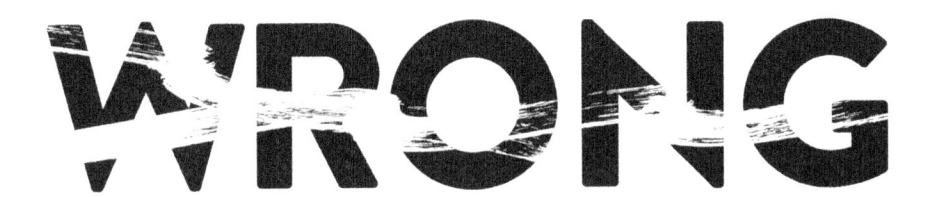

EVERYTHING THEY TOLD YOU ABOUT MENOPAUSE WEIGHT LOSS IS WRONG

**Everything They Told You About
Menopause Weight Loss is Wrong**

Second Edition, Copyright © 2025 by Ailsa Hichens

All rights reserved. No part of this book may be reproduced, stored in a retrieval system, or transmitted in any form or by any means—electronic, mechanical, photocopying, recording, or otherwise—without prior written permission from the publisher, except for brief quotations in critical reviews or articles.

Published by Eglantine Press

Paperback ISBN: 978-1-0683168-2-1
eBook ISBN: 978-1-0683168-3-8

This book is intended for informational purposes only. The author is not a medical professional, and the information provided should not be considered medical advice. Always consult with a qualified healthcare provider before making any changes to your diet, lifestyle, or healthcare regimen.
Any similarity to real persons, living or dead, is purely coincidental.

EVERYTHING THEY TOLD YOU ABOUT MENOPAUSE WEIGHT LOSS IS WRONG

AILSA HICHENS

CONTENTS

Introduction 7

PART ONE
Chapter 1 - How does your metabolism get broken? 17
Chapter 2 - Get back in control of your blood glucose 25
Chapter 3 - This is how weight loss works 35
Chapter 4 - Metabolism, calories, & hunger 43
Chapter 5 - Other metabolism wreckers 51

PART TWO
Chapter 6 - Metabolism boosting guidelines 63
Chapter 7 - Exactly what to eat 73
Chapter 8 - Foods that help you lose weight 87
Chapter 9 - How to eat 95
Chapter 10 - Make fasting work for you 107

PART THREE
Chapter 11 - Sleep, the real game changer 117
Chapter 12 - How to sleep better 127
Chapter 13 - Stress & your metabolism 137
Chapter 14 - Create an anti-stress action plan 145
Chapter 15 - The right exercise 155
Chapter 16 - Getting a bit more active 163

PART FOUR
Chapter 17 - Get your head in the game 171
Chapter 18 - Planning & prep 181
Chapter 19 - Actually doing the work 191

References 197
Resources 204
About the Author 205

INTRODUCTION

To say everything changes in the 'menopause years' is like saying it's a bit nippy in the Arctic. Maybe you have hot flushes, night sweats, you can't sleep for toffee, your 'downstairs' is like the Sahara, your memory and mood are shot - or one of scores of other punishing symptoms. Or you could be one of a gazillion women struggling to lose weight. Any which way, the problem is not you, it's your faulty midlife metabolism, and this book is all about fixing it.

Although this is not really a book about menopause and how to reduce your menopausal symptoms, in many ways it is. You're having a midlife metabolic meltdown (not an official term). When you understand why all this stuff is happening, you can play your hand in the very best way you can to get the health and the body you want.

Thankfully there's now an acknowledgement that menopause can be a huge deal for women*, impacting every area of their lives, from their health symptoms, their relationships, their work life and how it feels to be a woman* more generally. Not every doctor, employer, friend (or even the women themselves) are enlightened, of course, but things are much better than they were.

Hormone replacement therapy (HRT) - even if you do take it - is not going to save you. It may make a lot of things better, but you have to do the food, lifestyle, and movement work to get the kind of life you deserve. Any one of a number of things could be awry and I'll do my best to cover most of them in this book. This might be your first foray into trying to sort this out. Equally, I hear from women all the time who have really been tackling their menopause head-on and are still frustrated by their lack of progress.

This book is for *all* midlife women:

The serial dieter who restricts what she eats and has done so on and off throughout her adult life. She's done all the diets ever invented. She's always starting again on Monday and never really makes any progress.

The habitual calorie counter who eats really low fat and barely ever eats 'bad' foods. She's always been 'good' at dieting and following a plan to the tee but now progress has ground to a halt no matter what she tries. (By the way, we don't do 'good' and 'bad' here. It's terrible for your headspace and, anyway, no food is inherently good or bad, no matter what it is.)

The chronic exerciser who has taken the 'move more' ethos pretty close to the limit at times. Likely to be often indulging in frequent runs, spin classes or long cardio sessions designed to burn the maximum number of calories.

The busy, stressed-out exec that may or may not additionally involve any of the above.

The woman trying to juggle it all - work, family/ other caring responsibilities, relationship, social life, chores, and general life admin - and can only manage this all by extending her day and shrinking her sleep.

The woman jumping from test to test trying to find the answers because she recognises that data is power, but she still hasn't found the answer - although she's ploughed through a lot of cash doing so and has an impressive number of jigsaw pieces but can't fit them together yet.

I see all these scenarios in my nutrition clinic. It isn't your fault you aren't where you want to be. The public health message is decades behind real-time nutritional science, some health professionals are dinosaurs, and there are a lot of very shouty people on social media talking a load of bollocks. These days, everyone has an opinion (including me, so I do recognise the irony) so small wonder it's impossible to know who you can trust.

If we haven't met, let me introduce myself. My name is Ailsa Hichens. I'm a Registered Nutritional Therapy Practitioner. At the time of writing, I'm 52 and I'm pretty sure I'm post-menopausal though, with a coil, it's anyone's guess. As you might expect from someone with my job, I have a decent diet most of the time - although I am partial to rhubarb crumble and custard, trifle, and salt and vinegar crisps (not always together). Like many nutrition professionals, I gravitated towards professional training having spent years trying to fix aspects of my own health, geeking out on information about nutrition and then throwing my hat over the wall to study the thing for four years.

After years spent helping individual clients and groups and generally making a difference, you could say I was complacent about my own health. But then here's what happened…

My story

I'm going to make this pretty snappy. The point is, I've been there. I'm not a nutritional gnome sitting in her kale palace dishing out advice on circumstances I have not been through myself.

I'd had a rough eight years. Relationship stress, messy divorce, family dramas, home move, too much work, sudden bereavement, all of which impact on the healthiest of folk, but I had some underlying (but managed) complications, and the net result was all the stress, no me time, too much work, too much sitting on my arse doing said work, too little sleep. Perimenopause chaos.

I was a ticking time bomb though still ostensibly healthy. I didn't smoke, and I ate well nearly all of the time (although, admittedly, the wine sometimes crept above where it should have been but, hey, I was dealing with things, OK?) The weight was creeping on because of any one or all of the above. In truth, I felt like a bit of a fraud since I was privately wondering whether I was falling apart. Sometimes we need a wake-up call to get in action.

And this was mine. It wasn't anything huge; just the last nail in the coffin.

It was a routine appointment at the optician. I go every two years since I'm a good girl and they ask me to but also usually only to be given a stronger prescription for my reading glasses. I had all the tests and was expecting the optician to tell me how they had rarely seen such fabulous eyes - but there was trouble.

Cataracts forming in both my eyes. That's clouding in the lens in your eye that causes blurry vision and visual disturbances. Wait, what? Not serious, just the beginnings and, since it was the first time they had been spotted, the optician was not sure how quickly the downhill slide would be before they needed to operate. Ew, being awake while they cut my eyes. Hello, am I 80 or something? I was 51.

Obviously, I turned to Doctor Google to get the very worst-case scenario to fret over. Continued sight loss and eventual blindness. And that was the moment. The one that came after the toppy cholesterol warning, rising blood glucose, having half a wardrobe of clothes that didn't fit, looking very decidedly frumpy and middle aged in any photos I was unlucky enough to find myself in.

I didn't discover until much later that the early cataract business is hereditary but mostly those early signs in our family don't advance any further. But at the time I was spooked and, as the only living parent to my three children and four cats, I was panicked about what might be in my future if I didn't fix my sh1t as a priority.

That meant tidying up loose ends in my diet, actually doing the work on stress reduction, and getting enough sleep, making sure my gut was in a happy place and turning up the dial on the kind of exercise that was going to save my skin and my health.

If you're thinking, well, it's OK for her knowing all this stuff but what will I do? That's why I wrote this book.

I am not alone in this. Perimenopause and beyond makes life (and health) a lot more complicated and, since you picked up this book, one way or another you're wading in similar waters. I don't mean that you will necessarily have blood glucose problems but, in all honesty, there's a chance your metabolism needs a bit of a glow-up and now is as good as any time to get started.

Throughout this book, I'm going to be talking you through the basic science (don't worry, there won't be a test) because I find it's really helpful to know what your body should be doing so you can spot if it's gone awry.

However boo-hoo you might be feeling about your body and your health, let's not dwell since it will drag you under, which is the exact opposite of empowering. Let's not pine for past glories. Instead, I warmly invite you to take inspiration from a sign I have in my office… When I was at the highest point of misery following my divorce, one of my best friends bought me a card with (in my view) the *best* motto: 'Chin up, tits out, onward.'

Throughout this book you can count on me for this:
I promise you straight talk.

And an action plan. Some of this might challenge what you thought you knew. You might wonder how on earth you can possibly fit all this in. Don't worry, it's my job to help you work that out.

I want to assure you that we are not going on a knitted yoghurt-fest. You're going to be getting real-life solutions. When I work with my private clients, I make sure my programmes are designed for real women living real lives that are sometimes busy and messy and far from perfect, and they feature real food rather than the kind you can only get from health food stores. Yes, I will be asking you to do something different because if you do the same, you will get the same, right? But it will be manageable.

My goal for this book is that it becomes your midlife strategy. Not everyone will find everything directly relevant as we are all different, will have different symptoms, experiences, and lifestyles, but there will be something good you get from your reading this.

Here's what you will get from this book
You'll understand how and why things are different in your body in perimenopause, menopause and beyond. By that, I mean expect some talk about what happens to your hormones in midlife. When I say 'hormones', I'm not just talking about the obvious lady hormones like oestrogen, progesterone and even testosterone, but your hunger and satiety hormones, and those that directly regulate fat storage and fat burning.

You'll really get the 'new rules' for optimum metabolism in your 40s and beyond so that you can (with my help) create a strategy that fixes what you need fixed in your health.

You'll create a practical, highly do-able strategy for yourself that works in your actual life and that, rather than sounding like a punishment, feels like an exciting challenge.

You'll discover how you can easily make changes in your life that stick long-term - and that come from being clear on what you want, why it matters and how you're going to inevitably sabotage your good work (we're all human and we do weird stuff - it's normal).

I've tried to split the book up into a logical journey for you. The book is divided into four parts: why, eat, live, do.

Part one – Why? The biology of metabolism

In order to really take action and feel compelled to try something different, you will need to understand a teeny bit of the basic science. I really want you to get what is happening to your midlife body and, empowered by this knowledge, the 'what to eat piece' and the lifestyle advice then makes sense. So, in this section there are chapters on how your metabolism goes wrong as you age, why blood sugar balance is the solution you need, how weight loss actually works and the truth about calories in versus calories out.

Part two - What to eat

According to my family, I have always been a bit over-interested (their words) in what goes in and what comes out. As a Registered Nutritional Therapy Practitioner, it would be weird if I didn't talk about food, so I'll give you the best food strategy and tactics for this stage of your life. So, that's the deal about macros and micros (don't worry if these are meaningless for you right now, it will make sense later, I promise), foods that spike your blood sugars and how to avoid those spikes, and also foods that rev up your metabolism. Yes, there are some, but you cannot just skip to this chapter and ignore the rest because, while they will help you, they are not magic - you have to do the rest of the work or you're wasting your time.

I will give you lots of guidance on how to build meals and snacks that work for your midlife body, but this is not a recipe book. There are enough of those around. But you'll leave me certain of what to eat and why it matters, and I'll signpost you to some great resources.

Not eating also has its place as a midlife metabolism fixer. Most people eat too much and eat too often. Strategic not eating aka fasting is your secret weapon here - but you need to do it right. There are specific things that work for men that do not for women, so we'll be avoiding those. There are strategies that are right for younger women, and those that are better suited to women like you in their prime. So that's the kind we'll be talking about.

Part three - Lifestyle fixers

This part of the book is about the lifestyle aspects that make a difference. When I first qualified as a nutritionist, I used to think all that mattered was the food. Maybe it's because I wasn't menopausal back then. Now I know better.

First out of the blocks in this section is sleep. Why it matters and how to get more quality sleep. Seriously, if you are doing all the food work but you are not sleeping well or you are not sleeping enough, you will not get the results you want.

How you take care of stress and reward yourself is super important. As a woman over 40, your declining hormones mean that you are less resilient to stress - and that's why so many feel overwhelmed in perimenopause. Again, it is what it is, and it isn't what it isn't. The biological role of stress goes directly against what you are trying to achieve with your health but, after you've read this chapter, you'll have an action plan for taking back control. If you're reading and thinking, 'Stress, that's not me', consider that you don't need to be going through a divorce or a house move or have suffered a bereavement or even feel particularly stressed in order to *be* stressed; the constant and relentless drip, drip, drip of everyday life is enough.

Moving your body matters for lots of different reasons. I'm not a personal trainer so I won't be giving you a work-out plan, but it will be important to get moving or switch up your current routine to one that benefits rather than sabotages your midlife metabolism. So, there's a chapter dedicated to muscles and movement, and you'll want to be prepared to do some things differently now. Yes, it's another thing that will take some time but remember, right now is where you'll be creating your life for the health you want in your 50s, 60s and onwards.

Part four - How to do the work

This is where we start pulling it all together. It's all very well knowing what to do but usually more knowledge doesn't mean more action. So, the final section of the book is where you'll actually create your personal action plan. We'll look at finding your 'why' (which is code for why the hell it matters to actually do anything different since no one ever took an action without knowing 'what's in it for me?').

You'll work out how to get started, measure progress, keep going (because you know that, even if you start, you will eventually want to go back to 'normal' when it gets hard) and strategies for not mucking up all your progress.

We're not delving into all the other possible reasons your health is not the way you want it to be. There are other books (and who knows, maybe I'll find a second book inside me) to be written on thyroid health, detoxification, inflammation and so on, but we'd be here way longer than is strictly necessary.

I cannot wait for you to get started. I hope this sounds like what you need.

* I do recognise how people identify and choose to be classified has changed in the last decade and it is for brevity only that I write 'woman' and 'women'. If you are biologically a woman going through menopause, this is you. I don't want to over complicate my sentences or tie myself in knots so please, when you read 'woman', insert however you want to refer to yourself. The same for she and her. Apologies in advance, no harm meant with any of this. Can you be OK with that?

PART ONE

CHAPTER 1
HOW DOES YOUR METABOLISM GET BROKEN?

In your quest to lose weight over the years, you've probably had a view about your "metabolism". Maybe you were lucky and yours was fast. You could eat what you liked in almost any amount and not gain a pound. Or else you drew the short straw. With your slow metabolism, one look at a biscuit and the pounds were reluctantly added to your hips.

I've never been one of those skinny types with a zippy metabolism. Losing weight or maintaining it has been a complicated picture. I've been on every diet known to womankind and popped all kinds of pills in the name of speeding up my metabolism, including some from an especially dodgy office set-up down a dingy London alley that I'm pretty sure - looking back - were amphetamines.

Today, what I find in my nutrition practice is that most women in midlife have a 'problem' with their metabolism. Even if once you had the metabolism to challenge a shiny new Ferrari, now it resembles a clapped-out Lada. So here seems a good place to get clear on what your metabolism actually is, why it matters and what goes wrong from perimenopause onwards.

I must warn you, it gets a touch gloomy for a while. All your hormones go a bit haywire, and the chance of problems increases dramatically. But you have control over more of this than you think. I don't want it to be all miz and for you to give up reading before we get to the good and empowering stuff, but you do need to know some truths about what we midlifers are up against in the world of health.

So, put on your big girl pants, strap in, and let's push through the nasty stuff so we can get to the other side quicker.

Your metabolism is your body's motor

To carry on with the car analogy, think of your metabolism as your engine, your personal power plant fuelled by food and creating the energy your body needs to function at its best. Metabolism isn't just one simple process. It's a complex web of biochemical reactions happening all throughout your body. It encompasses a wide range of activities, from digesting and absorbing nutrients to getting rid of waste products. It's happening whether you're lifting weights at the gym or lounging on the sofa binge-watching Bridgerton.

This is a massive over-simplification but let's keep things on a need-to-know basis. In your twenties and thirties, everything works well. All the machinery is functioning as it should for your engine to be running at its best. You have bags of energy, you're much more likely to be at your happy weight, you're sleeping well and everything looks rosy.

Then along comes perimenopause. You know this already, but everything changes, and the root of it all is your faulty midlife metabolism. Fix this, and everything will start to come back into line.

This is how it all goes wrong over 40

As you enter your early to mid-forties, the hormonal fluctuations associated with the transition to menopause wreak havoc on your metabolic rate. Here's a snapshot of what's going on:

Declining oestrogen changes where you store your fat. Instead of storing it around the hips (hello hourglass), now extra weight congregates around the middle just like a man (what the hell, bowling ball).

Another hormone involved in fat distribution is progesterone. While oestrogen levels fall more gently in perimenopause, progesterone falls off a cliff. Progesterone has a balancing effect, helping prevent fat storage in the abdominal area. So, when progesterone levels decrease, the oestrogen-to-progesterone ratio shifts, favouring fat storage where you least want it.

The 'male' hormone testosterone is also needed by women albeit in smaller amounts, but levels decline with age, and this impacts fat distribution as well. Lower testosterone means a reduction in muscle mass, which lowers your metabolic rate (how much energy you use just to stay alive) and increases fat storage, particularly around your middle. Simultaneously, family and work commitments seem intense at this stage of life and often mean exercise and movement take a back seat, which makes the situation worse. No judgement - I found myself in this exact situation.

Declining oestrogen is also responsible for this enormously important piece of the puzzle: increased risk of insulin resistance. This is BIG and we'll go into this in detail in the next chapter. Let's just say, for now, you cannot handle the same number of carbs you could a decade ago. This is because many women lose their sensitivity to insulin, and this lack of insulin sensitivity is often what's lurking behind your midlife weight gain and many of the other irksome symptoms of menopause like hot flushes and sleep problems.

That fall in oestrogen impacts how well you sleep and also how well you cope with stress. Typically, women sleep less well and with more interruptions, and feel overwhelmed more easily than they did pre-peri. You can take whatever view on that you like, but this book won't dwell on what has been, we'll move forward powerfully and control the new era we are living into.

Of course, individual variations exist, and not all women will experience the same changes in fat distribution during menopause. Genetic factors, lifestyle choices, and overall health can also influence your metabolism. However, I'm betting at least some of this resonates already…

This book isn't a conversation about whether you should be replacing lost hormones with HRT. Most of these bothersome symptoms can only be fixed with food and lifestyle changes, and that is what we are talking about here. What we will be doing is lifting the lid on your car bonnet, getting out the tool kit and making some necessary adjustments so that your engine is firing on all cylinders again. (Sorry for all these car analogies. It is ironic that I'm using them since I am incapable of doing even minor maintenance on my car - like filling the screen wash or checking the tyre pressure.)

This is also a book for every midlife woman, even those who have sailed through perimenopause very nicely thank you and aren't aware there even is a (potential) problem. The majority of what I'll talk about does apply to you even if you haven't experienced any notable symptoms so far. Knowledge is power. There will come a time when this might become important...

Some quite depressing sit-up-and-take-note facts (sorry)

59% of women over 16 are overweight, obese or dangerously obese. That figure climbs to 73% of women aged 45-53, right in that menopausey zone.

These numbers have shot up in the last couple of decades and will climb further still if we don't do something about it. And by that, I don't necessarily mean governments should do something. I think women owe it to themselves to take responsibility for having a decent and health-filled future.

I don't say this to be the fat police but there is a correlation between health, disease and death and people carrying a lot of extra weight. If your Body Mass Index (BMI) in the high range (over 25 is overweight and over 30 is obese), you are at far greater risk of type 2 diabetes (which, although manageable and potentially reversible comes with some pretty nasty additional complications including sight loss and amputated limbs) and coronary heart disease.

The number of people in the UK with diabetes has topped 5 million and 90% of those have type 2 diabetes, which is a 'lifestyle disease' caused by food and lifestyle choices. If you're thinking, phew that's not me, lucky times, an estimated 850,000 people in England alone are sitting with the ticking time bomb that is undiagnosed type 2 diabetes. So it could be that it's all going on under the bonnet, but you haven't felt unwell enough to go to the doctor about something and had this discovered by testing.

Diabetes is not a place I want anyone to head to but, if you're a woman with diabetes, things look even more bleak. You're twice as likely to get heart disease as a man (and you have a lower chance of surviving a heart attack) and you have a higher risk for blindness. When you hear 'heart problems' you're probably imagining an older man or one with less-than-favourable food and lifestyle habits, right? And you'd be right, but the number one killer (after dementia and Alzheimer's) in women of menopausal age isn't breast cancer (although it gets a lot more column inches) but heart disease although this isn't really spoken about. While you might be unlucky as far as the Big C goes, you are twice as likely to be killed by heart problems. That's because, in your younger years, oestrogen has a protective effect on your heart. Low levels in midlife increase the risk of arteries narrowing and plaque forming. Narrowing of the arteries is also associated with stroke. There are other risk factors, too, outside of smoking and drinking in excess. I mentioned having diabetes already but add to this having high cholesterol and being overweight. All of these are more likely (but not inevitable) in women as they get older.

Before you say it, you can be pretty healthy and overweight and it is also the case that you can be skinny and super unhealthy. This is a broad brush. The overweight category will encompass people who aren't bothered by their weight, which is fine (this is a free country after all), but also people who deeply care yet have got overwhelmed or stuck trying to fix themselves.

This is relevant for you even if you think you lead a decently healthy life. It was me, too, a while back. I told you the tale of my optician visit in the introduction, but it is worth emphasising that it was a real wake-up call. As a nutritionist, I had a decent (but not perfect) diet although at the time I also probably drank a little bit more wine than I should. I could have done more exercise, which was tricky to fit in with a busy life and other priorities. I was likely on the healthier side of being a regular woman. And yet…

But wait, there's a LOT you can do about this

I appreciate this is very depressing reading but stay with me because I bring good news: the Interheart study (2004) followed 30,000 people in 52 countries and researchers found that lifestyle changes could prevent at least 90 percent of all heart disease. So just in case you're thinking this is your fate so why fight it, there is a lot you can do about it - and this is why I wrote this book.

I see women transform their health time and time again in my nutrition clinic. These are all regular women who have committed to making some reasonably straightforward changes. They're not special - although we are all, of course, special. I mean, they are no different from you and me. They are dealing with real life in all its messiness and yet still the magic happens.

I appreciate it seems like a lot to take in and often there are some initial questions people want answers to before we get into the details about how we're going to fix this thing.

This is not fair, why do men not have to deal with this?

I agree, it's a bitter pill, but it is what it is, and it isn't what it isn't. I'm going to be straight with you and say that you really have to move on and take control of the situation as it is to get the new you you're looking for. You cannot have success by sticking in victim mode. Besides which, it is the opposite of empowering and who needs that drain on their life?

Wait, you're telling me I can't have any carbs?

I'm not but - spoiler alert - you will not want to be eating the same ones in the same quantity as you are now and anyone who advises you otherwise at your stage of life is plain lying. Carbs are not the enemy, but they are not your besties any more. Don't worry, though, we'll work this through in the next few chapters.

This feels too complicated, I'm just going to carry on.
Surely what I'm doing will eventually work, it's just taking time.

Hmmm, we both know if you've been trying this for a year or more without success, it's not happening.

I get it, I'm just eating too much, and I need to exercise more.

Maybe but very possibly not because the calories in and calories out theory is [and insert own choice of bad word] and anyone who tells you this is likely to be one or all of these things:
- Not in perimenopause or menopause so have zero personal experience and probably won't be working with many perimenopausal women either;
- A man (sorry if you're an enlightened one among them but I see way too many poorly informed guys on socials talking b*llocks, telling people it is only about eating less and moving more);

- Trained *only* in dispensing exercise advice with no robust training in personalised nutrition.
- A personal trainer speaking to an audience of women who are lifting weights and do so very regularly, and who have a decent diet already. This is a different ball game altogether. We will talk about this calorie in v calories out business a lot, so don't worry but this is one thing I really want you to leave behind now you're in this phase of your life.

I'm obviously just meant to be this way.

If you can 100% truly, utterly, and happily accept the way things are with no wishes that things were otherwise, that's no problem. Except, you know that's not the case. You picked up this book because you wanted to change something. We can go at any speed you like. This is not a race, it is the rest of your life. You are literally designing the whole next chapter of your life - your future health - right now and I want to inspire you to create the very best version of yourself that you can.

That sounds like it should be on a poster.

> **10-second recap**
>
> In perimenopause, changing levels of the sex hormones oestrogen, progesterone and testosterone affect more than just your periods and cause typical symptoms of menopause like hot flushes, anxiety and brain fog. They wreak havoc on your metabolism, making you react differently to food, store more fat, and store that fat around your middle. You're also more likely to experience sleep disturbances and lose your resilience to stress, which, in turn, makes it more likely you'll weigh more. You're also at greater risk of other bad health events, so it is time to do something different. Food and lifestyle change are the medicine you need. It's not as hard as you expect. And there is less lettuce involved than you might think too.

CHAPTER 2
GET BACK IN CONTROL OF YOUR BLOOD GLUCOSE

There are all kinds of different things you can measure and rebalance in your health but, for midlife women, the starting point is blood glucose control since this is central to how efficiently your body works. I don't want to be overly dramatic, but this is the key to *everything*.

If you picked up this book because you want to lose weight, you're going to have to get your head around the fact that the diet industry has been lying to you for years. They convinced you that you must focus first on restricting food, slashing calories and maybe even chopping out whole food groups. Calories in versus calories out is a maths problem that doesn't stack up for sustained weight loss.

Instead, we have to get the biology books out. Understanding how your metabolism works might sound a bit dull but - indulge me with the car analogy again - when you have the owner's manual for your body, all kinds of stuff about your health and how you feel starts to make sense. Ultimately, this new knowledge will allow you to improve your menopausal symptoms, get more energy, feel better, look better, sleep better, and - joy of joys - start to lose your menopausal middle. The big bonus is you'll shore up your health for your later years so that you can live more of them symptom-free and feeling your best.

What is blood glucose control & why does it matter?
rolls up sleeves

When you eat a cheeseburger your body doesn't recognise the burger as it is and neither can it actually use the nutrition in the burger exactly as you're consuming it. First, it must break it down into constituent parts. We'll talk about this in detail in Part Two when we cover exactly what to eat. Let's just say for now, the meat patty breaks down into proteins (amino acids), the fat (in the burger and the cheese) into fatty acids, and the rest (the burger bun, the leaves, the gherkin and tomato) since they're all carbohydrates, into sugar units or glucose.

Bread, pasta, rice, potatoes, noodles, cous cous, broccoli, carrots - or any other fruit and veg for that matter - as well as pastry, sweets, cakes and cookies are all broken down by your body into glucose - whether it's actual sweet-to-the-taste sugar or not. Some foods contain more glucose than others. Foods that release their sugars quickly cause a spike in blood glucose levels. It's an oversimplification but a helpful one.

The reason this matters is because your body doesn't like to have any more than what amounts to about a teaspoon of sugar in your blood at any one time. When you *repeatedly and over time* have too much sugar in your blood, bad things can happen, including (but not limited to) increased risk of heart disease, inflammation, nerve damage, eye problems, thrush and athlete's foot, and, if your body is unable to remove the excess sugar because your metabolism is broken, welcome to type 2 diabetes. Thanks to the typical Western diet, these events are becoming increasingly common.

Blood glucose levels do go up and down through the day in response to what you eat, and lifestyle factors like exercise and stress. This is completely normal. You would expect a small blood sugar excursion after a meal and this is not a big deal.

Your body is designed to cope. It's the repeated pronounced spikes that cause problems in the long run. But it's worth keeping in mind, each spike leads to the excess glucose being stored as fat - the opposite of what most women want.

What spikes your blood glucose?

Whether an individual ingredient or a meal spikes your blood glucose depends on several factors, including whether it contains any fibre or protein, both of which slow down how quickly the sugars hit your bloodstream.

Some carbs are 'simple carbs' and these release their glucose very quickly. Others are 'complex carbs', taking longer to break down and providing longer-lasting energy. Typically, 'simple carbs' won't contain any fibre, which is why they break down so quickly - like white bread, croissants or a bar of chocolate, for example. 'Complex carbs' (like seeded wholemeal bread or sweet potatoes) contain more fibre, which takes your body longer to digest, so the sugars are released more slowly.

Your body has a mechanism for preventing your blood sugar levels from staying high and it looks like this: after you eat a meal, your pancreas starts releasing the hormone insulin, which takes the extra glucose you don't immediately need out of your blood and stores it away because too much sugar can be hazardous. First, it takes the glucose into the muscles and then the liver, where it's turned into glycogen (the storage form of glucose). Only a certain amount of glycogen can be stored at any one time. The remainder – if it's unused within 24 hours – gets turned into fat by the liver.

So, think of insulin as the fat-storage hormone. If you want to burn body fat and reduce the amount of fat you store, you need to make less insulin, which means you need to look at the type and the quantity of carbohydrates in your life and match this against a variety of other factors we'll cover later.

Too much insulin

If you are eating more carbs than your body can handle too frequently, your body will need to make a lot of insulin to shift that potentially dangerous glucose out of your bloodstream. And when your insulin is elevated too often, your body loses its sensitivity to it.

Try thinking of it like this: imagine you're in a long-term relationship and you want your partner to help out at home. When you first get together, all you'd have to say is 'Darling, would you mind putting out the bins?' (insert your own example if that works better for you) and the job would be done. After ten years in the relationship, things are a bit more complicated. It's not that the job isn't *ever* going to be done, but you might have to ask quite a few times before it is.

Imagine a similar thing happening inside your body. You eat a meal that contains carbs so the body produces insulin because it needs to manage glucose levels and ensure any extra is taken out of the blood. Over time, the receptors on the cells may have become overworked and don't recognise insulin has been produced, so the signal is sent again. More insulin. The result is that, to complete the same job and to remove the same amount of glucose, more and more insulin needs to be made as the cells lose their sensitivity.

This is called being insulin resistant and it's very common in midlife women due to declining oestrogen levels. Oestrogen is not just a sex hormone. This key lady hormone, which naturally declines in perimenopause, has a whole gamut of roles in energy and glucose metabolism, but here are some of the highlights that are important to midlifers:

- Oestrogen increases insulin sensitivity, giving you a measure of protection against diet-induced insulin resistance.
- Oestrogen has a key role in brain chemistry for a variety of reasons and there's a link between insulin resistance and Alzheimer's Disease. Small wonder that Alzheimer's is more common in women than men and is listed as the number one cause of death in women.
- Oestrogen encourages your body to burn fat for energy rather than store it.

A lack of sensitivity to insulin is often lurking behind some of the more obvious symptoms linked to menopause like hot flushes, exhaustion, and difficulty concentrating/ brain fog. The lack of sensitivity is something we want to fix because insulin resistance is really only a hop, skip and a jump to prediabetes and type 2 diabetes.

The flip side is, when you are sensitive to insulin, you stay slimmer, hot flushes are less common, as are night sweats, and bone health improves, while cravings vanish and you feel and look full of energy.

Metabolic flexibility. This is where we want to be but what is it?

Metabolic flexibility (some refer to it as being 'fat adapted') is the desirable destination we want to reach. It describes a situation 'under the bonnet' of your car in which your body can use either carbs or your own body fat for fuel and passes seamlessly between the two without a noticeable drop in energy, mood, or performance. It's the ability and ease with which you can flip your metabolic switch.

Like a hybrid car that works initially on electric when you're nipping around town but for longer journeys starts using the petrol tank.

Most people have enough body fat to power them for weeks should they be unable to eat for some reason. It's not a desirable situation but my point is you probably could last a long time on your body fat alone if only your system could tap into it. The tendency these days is towards metabolic inflexibility and, if this is you, you might experience getting severe cravings, or feeling weak, shaking, or fuzzy-headed if you've not eaten for a while. We've even invented the term 'hangry' to describe the irritability we feel if the gap between meals stretches too far.

How do I know if I have a blood sugar problem? Get tested.

You might be wondering, how can I tell if this is going on? Will I feel it? The answer is that maybe you will and maybe you won't. Perhaps you'll notice some of the symptoms I describe above, but most women will be completely oblivious to what's going on inside their bodies because, well, if you're not regularly testing and you're not superhuman, you would have no way of knowing.

One of the things I regularly hear when clients first come to work with me is they feel they are being driven by some kind of mysterious force to eat the kind of things they *know* they shouldn't be eating but they feel powerless to stop. That, my dear, is likely to be a blood sugar imbalance. If you eat breakfast and are starving an hour or so later, ditto. When you eat lunch and are almost crushed by the 3pm slump, ditto. These are all signs that you need to get this thing back in control.

You can choose to go by how you feel or you can get tested. These days there are all kinds of tests and devices available if you want to look into your metabolic health, which I suggest you do.

After a certain age, your doctor is probably going to be interested in your metabolic health in any case, and many practices offer basic well-women investigations that are likely to involve measuring your fasting glucose levels and something called HbA1c. That's a good start. If there are reasons you don't want to go to the doctor's surgery, you can also get these done privately pretty cheaply from home using a fingerprick blood test kit.

Fasting glucose is a measure of how much sugar is in your blood at a particular time and it's done before you have had anything to eat or drink. It's most likely you'll measure first thing, just after you've got out of bed and before having your morning cuppa or anything to eat.

It's a reasonable starting point since, after your evening meal, the ideal scenario is that - just through the act of being alive - your body will have used up most of the glucose you consumed for your evening meal, so the first thing in the morning reading should be nice and low. If it's not, you'll want to look deeper, and you might want to stump up the small investment (about £20) to get your own finger-prick blood glucose monitor to keep an eye on things. For advice on what to look for, see the resources section at the end of the book.

Blood glucose readings:
- Morning fasting glucose levels should be between **4 mmol/L and 5.4 mmol/L** (72 to 99 mg/dL) for non-diabetics.
- **5.5 mmol/L to 6.9 mmol/L** (100 to 125 mg/dl) may be indicative of prediabetes.
- **7.0 mmol/L or more** (126 mg/dl or more) may suggest diabetes.

If you are measuring your fasting sugar levels and get a reading you don't like, don't jump to conclusions. It could be a blip. If you have a few consecutive readings you don't like, make an appointment to see your doctor. There are a few things outside of food and drink that have an impact on blood glucose readings, not least stress and poor sleep.

However, this test is not the best indication of insulin resistance (which is what we really want to look into as a midlifer) because you're looking at a single data point – literally the time you pricked your finger. This is one reason why having your own glucose testing kit can be helpful, and it is also why many doctors are more interested in your HbA1c level.

Note: there are other tests but, in practice, fasting glucose and HbA1c are the two most commonly requested.

HbA1c stands for haemoglobin A1c and it's a measure of your average blood sugar levels over the past two to three months. It might be tested alongside fasting glucose by your doctor, but equally you can get this test done inexpensively yourself.

Haemoglobin is a protein found in red blood cells that carries oxygen to different parts of the body, and glucose has an affinity for it, which means it attaches to it, forming a 'glycated' haemoglobin molecule. This scientific union shows what's been happening over a longer period of time. It's a test I often recommend to my clients.

HbA1c Readings*
- **Normal**: below 42 mmol (under 6%)
- **Prediabetes**: between 42 and 47 mmol (6% - 6.4%)
- **Diabetes**: 48 or higher (6.5%) higher on two separate tests
- *Source: Diabetes UK

About continuous glucose monitors

I'm betting you've seen people on social media or around and about sporting a little white disc on their upper arm. It's a continuous glucose monitor or a similar device called a flash glucose monitor.

For some people, measuring blood glucose is a medical necessity. I'm thinking here of people who have been told they have diabetes and want to get back in control of their glucose levels or, for type 1 diabetes, they need real-time information to work out how much insulin they need to dose. Since very high sugars are dangerous to the body and very low sugar levels (hypos) can be life-threatening, these monitors can mean the difference between life and death.

The surge in popularity of these devices has come from their greater availability (and more marketing) for regular folk who are who are looking for answers as to why their energy levels are on the floor or why their weight loss efforts aren't working, or maybe they're the sort who love getting data on what their body is doing. Any reason is good enough as far as I'm concerned.

These monitors are great for providing real-time updates on what your body is doing through the day, either continuously (continuous glucose monitor or CGM) or with a little more input from the wearer by means of ensuring you hold your smartphone against the monitor every handful of hours (flash glucose monitor, which is the more common device). The term CGM is commonly used to refer to an actual CGM but also a flash glucose monitor so for brevity, I'll also refer to them as one and the same given the job they do is almost identical.

I'm not going to turn this into a giant conversation on what I think about CGMs. You'll find much more of that on *Notes from Midlife* blog at foodfabulous.co.uk. However, let me race you through some key points.

The lowdown on continuous glucose monitors

Do I think it's a good idea to wear one? Yes, probably, and likely for a couple of months, which will set you back a few hundred £££ because in reality, just getting one monitor lasting 14 days won't give you enough raw data. Even if you know what you're doing, it can take a while get your head around what the numbers actually mean for your life.

The data from your CGM is super interesting but you've got to know how to read it - otherwise it's a meaningless graph. Not all apps are created equal. Some literally just show you a few squiggles, which would be impossible to turn into useful information. Whether you're working with a coach like me to turn these numbers into your own 'magic formula' or trying to do this on your own, you *will* need a decent companion app that interprets this data and allows you to input your food and exercise so you can see how these affect your glucose levels. Find my recommendations in the Resources section at the end of this book.

For some people, this level of knowledge is not healthy. If you have an unhealthy obsession with the scales, knowing your blood glucose levels is going to be one extra thing to have a bad relationship with and to obsess over.

View your CGM readings as a general trend not the be-all-and-end-all. If you have any kind of health anxiety, a continuous glucose monitor is not going to be your friend. In fact, the opposite. Wearing a CGM in this instance will drive your anxiety and keep you in fight-or-flight stress mode. This in turn will push up your blood glucose levels, which further fans the flames of alarm. If this is you, do not buy a continuous glucose monitor.

It's natural for your blood sugar levels to go up and down for all kinds of reasons. Yes, with the food you eat but also with stress, lack of sleep (which is in and of itself a kind of stress) and exercise (another source of stress on the body but a positive one). My blood sugar spiked when I got to a particularly sad bit in the *Eddie the Eagle* movie (don't judge). And when I started getting sick with a cold, my continuous glucose monitor went into overdrive. My levels were through the roof. Had I not been wearing a monitor, I'd have been none the wiser and, in this instance, that might have been a good thing.

It's not everything. One thing rarely is. Just like HRT (hormone replacement therapy). A single thing is probably not going to give you all the answers you're looking for. If you're wondering 'should I wear a continuous glucose monitor to help me lose weight' or else 'will a CGM help me manage my menopause', the answer might be yes but it equally might be no. Wearing a monitor will give you *some* information but the human body is complex and it might be that you need a little more unravelling.

Other forms of testing - like blood, stool, or genetic tests - might be even more illuminating. And this is why you might see other nutrition professionals knocking CGMs. It's not that continuous glucose monitors are a bad idea but they might not be right for you.

Personal view: ultimately, knowledge is power. Do with that what you will. If you need support, I have a programme for that.

For now, let's take a look at how weight loss actually works in the next chapter.

> ### 10-second recap
> The food you eat gets broken down into different units your body recognises: protein, fats, and sugars or glucose. Eat too many things that turn to sugar and that sugar is released too quickly, glucose levels spike and your body stores the excess as fat. Your blood glucose levels are important not only for weight; they can also affect how you experience the symptoms of menopause like hot flushes and are a player in other health conditions, including cardiovascular health and cognitive wellbeing. These may not seem important now but heart attacks and Alzheimer's are big problems for women's health.

CHAPTER 3
THIS IS HOW WEIGHT LOSS WORKS

There are all kinds of different variables that impact your weight. You are totally unique. Your genetic make-up, your lifestyle and previous medical history are all players. Scientists call it biochemical individuality. Then there are your personal circumstances and your dietary preferences. That means there isn't a single way of eating that's right for everyone. However, there is a very excellent general framework when it comes to fixing your metabolism and losing weight over 40 because most of the work comes down to sorting out your chemistry and, therefore, your hormones.

Doing this one thing is astonishingly effective, and it's what this book is all about.

If you're now raising a quizzical eyebrow, let me tell you that the big secret the diet industry doesn't want you to know is that fixing your chemistry is the game changer you've been looking for all along - and not the miracle potions, patches and pills they've been peddling. That's because approximately 75% of what you eat, including what you feel driven to eat, is down to your chemistry.

We'll deal with the calories in v calories out theory later but suffice to say, it doesn't stack up - and certainly not for menopausal women however many shouty men talk about it on social media. There are various things at play and I will lay them all out for you in a way that makes sense.

What repeatedly comes up in studies is that low carb works as a strategy for maintaining and/or losing weight. Don't read into that you need to eat no carbs or go keto or zero fat and cut the calories, all of which are about deprivation and are unsustainable. What I want for you is that you find joy again in food, feel satiated not starving, and stop those crazy cravings that have you diving headfirst into the biscuit tin. The benefit of this is that you'll probably discover more energy than you thought possible, sleep better, your skin might look clearer, and your hormones will begin to get back on an even keel.

When you're eating less stuff that turns to sugar, it makes it so much easier to get your body in a position to shed weight.

This is how your body will break down fat

Let's keep in mind what you actually want to do. You want to burn the extra fat you have on your body. That body fat is made up of three fatty acids joined together with a sugary molecule called glycerol. To lose weight, you need your body to use up all the glucose in your bloodstream (its preferred source of fuel), liberate stored fat, and then break down this fatty structure so it can be used as energy.

But it can't do that if you're topping it up with glucose all day.

Your body is not designed to work on the amount of carbs we eat today (compared to how our grandparents used to eat, for example). There are 'essential proteins' your body needs to survive (these are called essential amino acids), and there are 'essential fats' (essential fatty acids) but there are no essential carbohydrates. Your body is perfectly happy to switch to using fat as a fuel but we rarely give it a chance.

In cavewoman times, your body would have alternated between using glucose and fats depending on the season. Some months of the year, you could fill your boots with berries and other plant-based foods (carbohydrates). When plants weren't available, you would have eaten a protein and fat-based diet as well as your own body fat reserves when food was scarce. This ability to switch between using these two types of fuel is called being 'fat adapted' or 'metabolically flexible' and it's a very desirable state to be in.

Centuries - and even generations - ago, a similar thing would have played out but today's modern diet is far higher in sugar and carbohydrates, and it's wreaking havoc with the world's health. Like most people, your body is likely to have become so used to relying on glucose for fuel that it has forgotten how to use (or rather, become unaccustomed to using) fat instead.

There are various reasons a low-carb diet (not no carb, remember) wins. It reduces cravings because you no longer have the huge spikes followed by troughs I discussed in the last chapter, and it keeps blood glucose moderate, allowing you to get more easily into a place where you can burn fat. Low carb is a way of eating that allows you to become metabolically flexible, regaining the ability to quickly and efficiently use both carbs and fat for food interchangeably and without crashing.

This is metabolic gold.

I'm not going to tell you you can't eat starchy carbs or sugar ever again. POV: the world is a poorer place without birthday cake and quiche. But you may need to cut back a bit (we'll get to this shortly) so your body regains that metabolic flexibility. If you're currently struggling with hot flushes and other menopausal problems like sticky weight gain, you have likely lost your metabolic flexibility. When you follow the guidelines set out in the book, you will be able to get back in control. Hurrah.

Years of crappy science and Big Food are stealing your health

A ton of bad science in the 1950s and the subsequent anti-fat propaganda pushed diets away from healthy fats and increasingly towards people filling up on bread, pasta, and rice. And the food industry has since been encouraging us to eat fat-free and, to fill the inevitable void, snack between meals - and often not on the 'right' things.

Without sounding like I'm a hundred years old, it just wasn't a thing when I was growing up for people to eat between meals, and you'd never have seen anyone walking down the street scoffing a sausage roll.

The good news is, your body can be re-trained pretty easily, and I'll show you how.

Back to my tale about using up your body fat...

Your body is more than happy to power itself on your fat but only when it has depleted the stores of glucose. When it does that, *that* is weight loss.

There is an element of truth in the calorie restriction theory but, in midlife, we both know there is something else going on because you already tried half-starving yourself and it got you nowhere. I think it would really help if you understood how these pieces fit together. I know, it's like GCSE biology all over again. I'm so sorry. Hang in there, you're doing brilliantly.

How the fat loss process happens is via a hormone called glucagon. Like insulin, it's made in the pancreas and its role is to stimulate the liver to release the storage form of glucose so your body maintains normal blood sugar levels. It can also command your fat tissue to release stored body fat to be used as energy.

So you'd want to make sure you're doing all you can to activate glucagon, right? What you also need to know is that insulin (the fat-storage hormone) and glucagon (the fat-burning hormone) are antagonists. Think of a light switch. It's either on or off. Where insulin is in the on position, glucagon is in the off position and vice versa.

You're either doing one or the other.

Most people spend a *lot* of the day eating. We are a nation of snackers. And, if you follow the nutritional guidelines set down by many government bodies who should know better (or, in fact, any of the big slimming clubs), your diet is likely to be 60+% carbs so you're practically stockpiling so much spare glucose, you never come close to running those stores down except perhaps in the middle of the night. At that point, you're nearly at a place to start losing… But then comes toast for breakfast, so forget it!

Midlife complications

Menopause puts a teeny spanner in the works. Years of overeating carbs (not your fault – you were probably just following the crappy dietary guidelines) plus various other lifestyle factors cause body fat to accumulate in the liver, and this eventually results in your body losing its insulin sensitivity. In other words, you become insulin-resistant. Then, even those things you think of as 'healthy carbs' like fruit and wholegrains can start to make you put on weight. We talked about that in the last chapter.

Sleep, stress, and movement are also important to this blood sugar/weight loss scenario. We'll talk about those in detail in part two of this book. For now, suffice it to say, lack of sleep, unchecked stress levels, and hardcore exercise schedules are further villains in this tale.

Here's how weight loss works in a nutshell

1. **Have less glucose available** in the body by eating less sugar and starchy carbs. You definitely won't want to do this by radically cutting back on calories or moving more because your body slows down to adjust to the reduced intake and you get hungry and miserable. To be clear, you don't always need to eat fewer calories to lose weight, but you do need to get less of them from carbs.

2. **Make less insulin**. Do this by eating fewer carbs and also by eating less often than you might have been told to do – and less often than you might be used to. If you eat breakfast, snack, lunch, snack, dinner and maybe a little something in the evening, you are topping up with fuel the whole time. When does your body get a break, let alone a chance burn off that fat?

   To lose weight, you need to spend as much of the day as you can not eating (but what's important here is that you are not radically cutting the amount of calories so your body doesn't run the risk of going into starvation mode). You also want to do this without triggering a rise in stress hormones, so don't go crazy with your fasting or Time Restricted Eating (more later). It's a tricky hormonal balance.

   Ideally, eat no more than three or four times a day, giving your body plenty of time to rest, repair, and reset in between. That's three meals and a snack if you need one.

   Don't panic! That might seem like an impossible challenge right now if you have been riding the sugar rollercoaster. Don't overthink it. If you follow the guidelines in the next chapters, it's going to be pretty easy.

   It is also helpful to time your meals so you have at least 12-14 hours between your last meal of the day and your first meal of the next day. You can achieve this by having dinner earlier (ideally) or breakfast later, whichever works with your schedule. We'll talk about fasting in a bit.

3. **Activate glucagon.** Switching on glucagon is harder than switching on insulin (where all you have to do is eat something). You can switch the fat-burning hormone on by running down glucose and insulin levels so it needs to find energy elsewhere. You can also do this by increasing your body's need for fuel – by moving. That doesn't need to be hardcore

exercise. In fact, for women over 40, lots of very high-intensity exercise is just too much for the body to take without flooding it with unhelpful stress hormones that keep blood sugar levels high. You need to build muscle for metabolic wellness (more of that later) as a priority as well as other types of movement for cardiovascular fitness and flexibility.

Sharon's story

Sharon came to see me because, while she was doing really well with her exercise regime, she felt she wasn't in control around food; her cravings were through the roof, her brain felt constantly foggy, and she felt the 'numerous chocolate bars' she was eating every day were sabotaging her otherwise healthy life.

Within two weeks of just changing her diet, she told me this:

"I already feel like a different person. I don't have as much brain fog. I can walk away from the Quality Street tin. I wasn't expecting things to have happened as quickly as they have. I have been mind-blown. And it has almost felt effortless."

It's at this point in many a book that you'll discover the person in question was eating kale stew and other weird foods. Not Sharon and, in fact, not any of my clients.

There's no need to eat anything you don't like or that comes from specialist shops. Sharon was eating Weetabix or porridge for breakfast and had simply made some tweaks to her regular meals. Importantly, she was low carb, and her body quickly responded.

10-second recap

To lose weight your body needs to use up the glucose it has in your bloodstream. Then it will look for glucose in your muscles and your liver, before finally tucking into your fat stores. The fat that gets liberated from your stores and then used is the amount of weight you will lose. Foods that contain less glucose and/or release that glucose less quickly make it easier for your body to do this work. You'll see later how lifestyle plays a role – muscles are glucose sponges and there are some lifestyle aspects (like stress and lack of sleep) that keep glucose high regardless, but we'll come to these later in the book.

CHAPTER 4
METABOLISM, CALORIES, & HUNGER

"The only answer to losing weight in midlife is to eat less and move more."

Never have so few words caused so much misery for so many and contributed so generously to misfiring metabolisms.

Of course, it does matter how much you eat, but calories matter far less than you think. What matters more is what you eat, oh, and the other stuff - how well your metabolism is working, how much sleep you're getting, how stressed you are, and all kinds of ancillary factors. And whether you're actually eating enough.

Eat less, move more, is a big, fat, dangerous oversimplification and is not supported by obesity researchers. Most importantly, it's way off the mark for us menopausal marvels.

Weight loss is very different for men and women and - I know you've worked this out already for yourself - everything is different from perimenopause onwards. A decade or more ago, if you wanted to drop a dress size for a holiday or an important event, you could simply skip a few meals, eat cabbage soup, hit the gym a little harder or, if you were really serious about it, do all of the above at the same time.

I see a great many women in my private clinic who are genuinely eating (with no misreporting) fewer than half the number of calories their body needs and yet the number on the scale has not dropped for over a year. Cutting calories has not provided the answer they were looking for. It never could and here's why.

This is what's wrong with calories in v calories out as a concept

It's the single biggest diet con ever based on a giant misunderstanding of the Laws of Thermodynamics. If you're interested in the science of this, I've tried to make it pretty straightforward to understand. If you just want to trust me on this point, skip ahead to the next chapter.

If you've chosen to hang in with the science, thank you. In the interests of preventing you from nodding off, these are some things I think you should know about it all:

- A calorie is the amount of energy needed to increase the temperature of 1 gram of water by 1°C.
- The calorie as we know it from food labels was introduced by scientist Wilber Atwater in late 1887. He worked out 1g of carbohydrate or protein provided 4 calories compared to 1g of fat providing 9 (you can start to see already how eating less fat compared to other foods might seem attractive). It's a figure that's still used today to calculate the energy you get from food.
- 19th century researchers believed a calorie was a calorie and nothing more, providing the same energy no matter the food. (Some people haven't moved much further than this even now - just saying.) This the First Law of Thermodynamics but it wasn't designed to measure anything other than mechanics - certainly not human biology.
- The Second Law (the Law of Entropy, since you ask) states some energy is lost doing 'the work'. Since this Law was developed during the Industrial Revolution, the 'work' probably involved heavy machinery but, when it comes to actual humans, it's subsequently been discovered that the act of eating and processing food also uses up energy so, while you might eat, say, 2000 calories in a meal, not all of them are retained as the body uses some of them up digesting the said meal.
- From the 1950s, an assortment of studies showed you use less energy digesting a meal heavy on carbs because carbs are really easy for your body to process, so more calories are retained. Conversely, the more protein or fat the meal contains, the fewer calories remain to be absorbed because the body has to work harder to process them.

In short, there's a difference between the calories retained when you eat broccoli compared to the calories retained from a chocolate bar.

Do calories matter at all?

They do *kind* of matter but calories are not the most important thing about eating, which is what many would have you believe. If you eat too much of anything, you will gain weight. How much you need to eat will depend on factors including your activity level but also on a variety of other just-as-important factors. This reliance on only counting calories as the best way of controlling your weight is deeply flawed since it's not the calories specifically that are the problem, it's your hormones.

Calories are not created equal and all calories do not cause weight gain. This has been demonstrated in a number of giant studies in the UK and North America.

Losing and gaining weight is about hormones, not just numbers. There are hormones that control your hunger levels and tell you you're full, and these are huge, which you will know if you have ever slashed your calories and relied on sheer willpower to get you through the day. Different hormones also regulate whether - and where - you will store fat.

You'll need to eat less - forever

This next bit is *big* for all seasoned dieters. Many diets - especially those you tried a decade or two ago - will initially have yielded great results but there's nearly always a price to pay further down the line by way of metabolic dysfunction. That debt is being called in now.

When you decrease the calories you put into your body, you also accidentally decrease the calories you use. This has been proven over and over in scientific studies. One of the most famous dietary studies ever published was by a man called Ancel Keys in *The Biology of Human Starvation* in 1950 and was based on a study of 36 healthy American men who were offered the chance to participate in the study rather than go off to war. They were monitored for three months to figure out roughly how many calories they needed to sustain their weight. Then they were starved for six months while still keeping up with their exercise regime (45-60 minutes of walking each day). This was followed by a period of three months during which the researchers gave groups of men different calorie and macronutrient meals to bring them back to good health. After that, they had a further two months of eating pretty much what they pleased. Just so you know, the 'starvation' phase saw them have their calories restricted to 1,570 calories, which is usually significantly more than some of my clients are eating each day when they first come to work with me.

There were a few interesting take-away points. First, many of the men concluded that going off to war might have been the easier option than this diet malarkey. They were always hungry, and reported weakness, dizziness, muscle wasting, fatigue, depression, irritability, a lack of coordination and their sex drive vanished. They also became totally obsessed with food and what they were or weren't eating. It's called 'semi starvation neurosis'. Does any of this sound familiar?

The study also showed that the more you cut calories, the more you need to keep cutting to sustain weight loss. When the men were into the eat-what-you-like phase, things didn't look pretty. It seemed their bodies would do anything to reverse the effects of the starvation. In those last couple of months, all the men binged (presumably to claw back some of those calories they had missed) and some just couldn't feel full no matter how much food they ate. The end result was that they gained not only all their original weight back but they increased their starting weight by 10%.

A huge study in 2006 (called *The Women's Health Initiative Dietary Modification Trial*, if you must know) looked at 50,000 postmenopausal women, dividing them up into two groups. One group was told to eat less and move more, the other was told to just continue as they were. After a whole year, the first group (who consumed 342 fewer calories each day by cutting down on fat) had lost an average of 4 pounds. Not much for such a sacrifice. The year after, they regained that weight and, when the study finished up after seven and a half years, there was no difference between the two groups. Not a single pound had been lost. There's more… In the first group, waist and hip measurements had actually increased so, although they didn't weigh more, they were fatter.

This is exactly what has likely been happening throughout your life when following diets you thought were doing you some good. Sure, the first few times you dieted by cutting calories, you lost weight in the short term but you likely regained it later and with interest.

Here's another thing to know: as a response to cutting calories, you are actually programmed to feel hungrier hormonally (and not just because less food is going in) and less satisfied by the food you eat – and that feeling of insatiable hunger can last long after you return to normal eating.

It's a repeating pattern. Cut calories, feel hungry, metabolism slows down, get obsessed about how much or little you're eating, meanwhile you need to eat even less after the diet to stay at a stable weight, get fed up or can't stand the deprivation, go back to eating normally, gain weight, start to cut calories again... and on and on it goes.

It's your hormones and nothing to do with willpower. Your body is literally compelling you to eat more food to survive. When you eat less, you feel hungry. You also have less energy and want to do less. And if you do more, you also get hungry and, unless you eat, you'll have less energy. You cannot win at this!

An inability to lose weight is not because there is something wrong with you, it's because of bad advice based on some shaky scientific assumptions. It's a fail on every level imaginable, not only because it doesn't work but because people we trust (the doctors and other health sources) tell us it should, and then we feel a big fat failure ourselves when it doesn't. So then you top feeling hungry with frustration with yourself for not being able to stick to a diet long enough, you develop anxiety around certain foods, lose confidence in your own body, and feel generally overwhelmed about what to eat since nothing you try actually works.

This is a common scenario I see in my nutrition clinic. If this is you, don't worry because your metabolism can heal from this.

You can't just move more either

If you lead a sedentary lifestyle, this is terrible for your midlife metabolism. Exercise is key for metabolic wellness, for your mood, your immunity, and your health in general but we'll come to that later in the book. What won't work for you is doing a lot of cardio, which tends to be what happens to women when they have their mind set on losing weight. They don't lift weights because they don't want to get bulky, and besides, they know running, spending hours on the elliptical trainer or Stairmaster, or taking a spin class will burn through more calories, and that's what they're trying to do to go down a dress size or two.

Exercise is important when it comes to fixing your metabolism and losing weight but it is not equally important. What you eat matters significantly more, and it's been shown over the years repeatedly that exercising more to lose weight brings consistently disappointing results.

My experience working with women is that, when it comes to weight loss, committing to an exercise programme is a signal to yourself that you are ready to take things seriously. You are in the zone. But to rely on exercise alone as a way to shed weight is an error. Of course, there is some impact but it is not as much as even the scientists testing the hypothesis had hoped.

One well-known large-scale study - *The Women's Health Study* - looked at three groups of women, dividing them into those who did a lot of exercise, those who did moderate amounts, and those who did little. Over the ten years the study ran, there was no noticeable difference in the intense exercise group compared to the others, and nor was there a change in body composition when it came to fat levels. Muscle was not simply replacing fat. This is a disappointment for many who put in hours at the gym hoping for a miracle. It simply demonstrates that you cannot out-run a bad diet. And yet moving your body in a way that feels good is important for health in general so don't cancel that class you have booked.

Exercise affects your desire to eat

If you've ever stepped up your workout schedule, chances are you've also eaten more or at least wanted to. What you're up against is the fact that the hunger hormone ghrelin spikes after a workout, while leptin (which tells the brain that you're full) plummets. It's a cruel injustice that this is peculiar to women. It doesn't happen in men. After a workout, women often eat more, which puts them at risk of gaining weight - the exact opposite of why most women exercise - but men don't have the same hormonal experience. Researchers are not sure why this is the case but speculate it might have something to do with biological programming to avoid energy deficits and preserve fertility so as to perpetuate the species since chronic undernourishment in women suppresses ovulation and hormones needed to reproduce.

So what really matters is what you eat?

Yes. And how you eat.

Most qualified nutrition professionals would say don't worry about the calories provided you are eating a 'good' diet (and I realise this is conceptual, but we will come onto this later in *What To Eat*). After all, it's impossible to accurately calculate how many calories *you* are getting from a specific food thanks to genetics, gut bacteria and the like, let alone what your body will do with those calories.

> ### 10-second recap
> Please stop believing that weight loss is just about calories in v calories out. The people telling you this are not writing about you. That stuff really mattered in earlier decades but it's a different ballgame now. Eating less may also be killing your metabolism.
>
> Exercise is important but less so than you think and maybe the 'right exercise' is also not what you think. What you eat matters, and how you eat.

CHAPTER 5
OTHER METABOLISM WRECKERS

The body is a complicated piece of kit and there could be all kinds of things going on with your health, so of course I am taking a big brush when I tell you all this. We've covered the biggie when it comes to metabolism, and that's glycaemic control aka blood glucose balance, but there are a handful of other things that might be relevant to this midlife mayhem you are experiencing.

Is your internal motor on go-slow?

The thyroid – a butterfly-shaped gland in your neck – is your body's internal motor, effectively setting the speed at which your body works. If it's not up to scratch, you might experience a whole host of uncomfortable or annoying symptoms. The hormones it makes affect most cells by increasing your basal metabolic rate, as well as dialling up heat production (in this case, a good thing and nothing to do with hot flushes). That's why people with an underactive thyroid often struggle to lose weight, feel the cold more easily and have low energy – imagine a record player playing a record at reduced speed… That.

Your thyroid can go wrong at any point but it's most likely you'll be diagnosed following childbirth or in your 40s because at these points you are experiencing the greatest hormonal storm and most likely to be bothered enough by the symptoms to trot off to the GP and get tested. There is also a complicated relationship with your thyroid, oestrogen, and menopause in general. In fact, thyroid symptoms can mimic menopausal symptoms so if any of the following resonate, you should ask your doctor for testing or better still, since routine testing will frequently only test Thyroid Stimulating Hormone (TSH), see a practitioner who can offer a full panel of thyroid tests that can pick up subclinical thyroid problems.

- Do any of these sound familiar?
- Feel tired all the time
- Hands and feet are always cold
- Putting on weight for no reason
- Can't seem to lose weight whatever I do
- Often constipated
- My muscles ache
- Get muscle cramps more often
- Feel irritable
- Generally, feeling a bit low
- Periods are heavier than usual
- Hair and skin feel so dry
- Sex drive is flagging or non-existent

Do you see how many of these overlap with the symptoms of perimenopause? It's worth knowing when you go to the doctor's surgery that what might be 'wrong' with you is perimenopause but it could also be an underperforming thyroid.

We could be here till Christmas with me talking about the thyroid but, in the interests of brevity, there are a few things you must know in order to have empowering conversations about your thyroid and your health.

Doctors - in the UK at least - will frequently only test Thyroid Stimulating Hormone (TSH) levels. TSH is the hormone that tells your body to produce the actual thyroid hormones. If your TSH is within range, your doctor is unlikely to run any further tests on the assumption that the rest of the hormone-producing cascade is working correctly. (As a side note, you'd be astonished how much your TSH needs to be off before anyone is even slightly interested).

If TSH is raised, your body is working harder than normal to produce the right levels of thyroid hormones. At this point, your doctor may repeat the TSH test in a few months to compare levels. Alternatively, they might test your Thyroxine (T4) levels to determine whether you're producing the right levels of this hormone. And that is where mainstream tests end.

If your T4 level is below range (or, in the case of an overactive thyroid, above range), indicating an underactive thyroid, you'll likely be prescribed a synthetic form of the hormone (thyroxine) to supply the body with what it is not making itself. It's not the ideal scenario, as you'll see in a moment, but if your T4 is low, you may feel better by taking thyroxine.

Even if your numbers 'look normal', if you're still dragging yourself through the day you could have subclinical thyroid problems. Depending on which country you're in, blood ranges for thyroid hormones are quite broad, so it's easy to fall outside the limits and have a thyroid that is not working quite as it should but it's not yet a disaster. Add to that, the whole thyroid hormone production is a cascade. If you're only testing one thing, this doesn't give the full picture of a complicated process.

Some people produce enough TSH and T4, but T4 isn't the hormone that actually does the work. Triiodothyronine (T3) is the 'work horse' that needs to be converted in the liver from T4. Some people, for various reasons, simply don't convert it very well. In other cases, you might produce enough TSH, T4 and T3, but the body negates the effects of the usable T3 by making reverse T3 (rT3) – literally reversing the action of T3.

If you're reading this from the UK, it's worth knowing that regular testing does not cover T3 or rT3, so if you're still feeling below par, it's worth getting a full thyroid blood screen done privately. (I can help).

And, in other important news, if you've been hoping that a prescription for levothyroxine was going to magically fix your broken midlife metabolism, it won't. Just like HRT won't solve all your menopausal woes, even if you can take it. Pharmaceutical drugs can be helpful and, in my experience, they can give you an initial boost, but they are never enough to feel on top of your game. You have to do the food and lifestyle work as well. There is no magic pill.

Your digestive health matters - even if you don't have tummy problems

If you've been suffering with digestive problems of any kind, you will know how important gut health is. If you don't (and I appreciate it's hard to be interested in something that doesn't feel that relevant to you right now), take it from me, it does really matter and here's why.

What's going on in your digestive system impacts your mood, energy levels, weight, hunger, skin, hormones (hello, hot flushes), and even how well you fend off illnesses. Believe it or not, your gut health can even have a say in how your lady bits behave. If you struggle with problems like irritable bowel syndrome, there's that, too.

It's all to do with the microbiome, a bustling ecosystem inside you, teaming with 100 trillion microbes. We call these gals the 'microbiota,' and they consist of bacteria, viruses, yeasts, and fungi, mostly hanging out in your gut.

Over the last decade, the science in this area has exploded and researchers have discovered an imbalance in the parallel universe that is your microbiome has far-reaching consequences for everything to do with your health. You might not know it or even feel it, but a good gut environment is the very foundation of health.

cue dramatic music

As you get older, the makeup of this ecosystem changes. Scientists can even pinpoint how old you are from the array of bacteria you have. Essentially, what happens is the bacteria become less diverse as you age and some of the most important – like lactobacillus and bifidobacterium – diminish in favour of more opportunistic bacteria ('bad' bacteria) and it's this imbalance that is often lurking behind unpleasant health symptoms.

Although researchers have long suspected the microbiome might hold the answer to the development of brain diseases like Alzheimer's, now they know for sure it does. There is a definite link between the type of bacteria in your gut and development of the disease. Since Alzheimer's is the biggest cause of death in women - as well as that complete loss of self being something most fear - if you want to hold onto your marbles, you must take care of your microbiome.

It turns out, your hormones and the microbiome are best friends. The 'estrobolome' describes the community of bacteria responsible for keeping your oestrogen levels in check. Your gut's bacterial balance can affect your sex drive, and those troublesome menopause symptoms like hot flushes, and night sweats. And, let's not forget 'downstairs'... Your vagina ages faster than you can imagine. In younger days, tightness was something you might have welcomed but in perimenopause, this can become problematic. Your vagina is the Thumbelina of body parts, and it literally shrinks and shrivels with age. The shrinking is technically called 'shortening', but it's a misnomer, and can make penetrative sex painful, especially when coupled with the bonus vaginal dryness that comes with this phase of life. This whole ladybits business is called vaginal atrophy - and the dictionary definition of 'atrophy' is 'partial or complete wasting away'. Brutal.

Much of the action in your digestive system is down to an enzyme called beta-glucuronidase, which affects the level of oestrogen circulating in the body and can result in too much or too little circulating oestrogen as well as changes in the various different forms of oestrogen. While the scientific community once thought menopause-related symptoms were just about the ovaries but now we know the gut plays a key role. The balance of oestrogen and progesterone affect the hormone receptors in your gut and this in turn governs how well (or otherwise) your gut works. An unbalanced gut is bad for menopausal symptoms.

But how does it mess with your metabolism?

Digestive issues have a big impact on how your body digests and absorbs food. While poor absorption can lead to weight loss, there are circumstances in which the gut environment can result in your piling on the pounds instead.

If you have Irritable Bowel Syndrome (IBS), the chance of you having a bacterial imbalance in the small intestine is very high. Many IBS sufferers do and it's officially called Small Intestinal Bacterial Overgrowth. If you're starting to think about 'good' and 'bad' bacteria, stop. In the small intestine, you don't want any bacteria because these bacteria compete with you for food. When they break it down, they ferment it, causing either hydrogen, methane or hydrogen sulphide gases. We'll not go into too many details here and, if you experience the symptoms of IBS (ranging from bloating and gas, to nausea, constipation or diarrhoea), it's worth exploring this further.

For now, suffice to say, bacteria in the wrong place can affect the overall function of the small intestine, allowing the lining of the intestine to absorb more calories from the food you eat as well as changing aspects of your metabolism, like affecting insulin and leptin resistance (leptin is the satiety hormone, which regulates how full up you get and it also signals your body to use stored energy). While it's important to have good diversity of bacteria in the gut, some strains appear more important than others for metabolic health. One of the key players is Akkermansia muciniphila, which - when abundant - is linked to better metabolic function or better glucose management, insulin sensitivity, less fat storage, and the reduced risk of cardiovascular disease.

So what does that mean for you in real life?
If you're already thinking of Googling Akkermansia in the hope you can pop a pill and beef up this area of your gut, thus getting your weight back on track, I don't recommend it. While you can buy this stuff in a bottle, gut experts question the efficacy of this kind of approach. Instead, the very best way to increase your levels is by growing a good gut environment with a polyphenol-rich diet, and we'll look at how in part two of this book. Besides, while research into specifically supplementing this bacteria looks promising, it's early stages and scientists warn of potential problems of supplementation in people with inflammatory bowel disease, polycystic ovary syndrome (PCOS) and endometriosis. Also of note, Akkermansia has been found to be raised in people with Parkinsons. Always err on the side of caution.

Once again, there is no magic pill and there is no shortcut. I'm so sorry. Stop trying to cheat. Is it annoying that your body seems to have a mind of its own and is on course for self-destruct? Hell yes.

This is, as you already know, not another diet book. It's designed as the instruction manual for your midlife body. In order to change your body and how it feels to be you, you need to understand how your body works so you can make the best decisions more of the time and get the health you want. You cannot simply take a bunch of pills to get there.

But it *is* possible to do something about it and I will be giving you a solid action plan. For now, I want you to know more about how your body could be playing up at this stage of life so that you are empowered to change.

It's all in your genes (well some of it, anyway)

We are all perfect and unique in our own way, and part of that is down to our genetic makeup. Your genes might set the path for certain diseases but this path is not set in stone. Very often, diet and lifestyle factors can influence those genes. Simply, by making different choices, you can change the course of your health - if only you knew which way your genes were pointing.

In this age of biohacking, it's possible to collect data on all kinds of aspects of your health and that includes your genes. If you have already done all the other stuff, sure, go ahead and find out how your genes are looking. If you haven't already taken the steps I'm going to be sharing in this book, my advice is start with the basics like blood glucose balance. Your genes are next level.

There's little point knowing you have a SNP (said 'snip' aka single nucleotide polymorphism, a variation or a change from the norm) that points towards a certain outcome if you're still eating sugary cereals for breakfast and a sandwich for lunch. But, if you've already done the food and lifestyle work, knowing which way your genes are pointing can be very helpful and a DNA panel focused on hormones and your metabolism or even your nervous system or thyroid, coupled with the right interpretation of your results, could make all the difference. I run a lot of these tests in my clinic.

There's no reason for you to have heard of any of these genes - most of my clients haven't until I suggest they test, but there are some that can explain many of your diet struggles.

You might learn, for example, you have two high-risk copies of the Fat Mass and Obesity Associated Protein gene, which was one of the first genes discovered that had a link with obesity. It's often referred to as the 'Fat Controller' or FATSO gene. This gene promotes the hunger hormone ghrelin and inhibits leptin, which tells you you're full and to stop eating, so you are likely to feel hungrier and eat more, and often seek out the classic high-carb Western diet of sugar, fat, and starchy carbs in your quest to feel fuller. You are more likely to weigh more and have a lower resting metabolic rate. In fact, it's the most important variant to know about when it comes to body weight.

Perhaps you have the 'Labrador' gene, named for the dog breed known for overeating. They're never satisfied even when they have just polished off a big bowl of chow because they genetically make fewer appetite-suppressing hormones.

There are, of course, some beneficial genes that can be manipulated - like the SIRT or FOX03 genes - that dial up the fat burning pathway and, if you knew how to do that, it might be useful…

You can also learn whether fasting is a good idea for your unique makeup, whether your body is programmed to love the high-fat ketogenic diet and other data that can help you build up a personalised nutrition and lifestyle plan.

Or you could discover you are super-quick to make stress hormones and need to put a self-care plan high on your list of actions to support weight loss in midlife.

The bottom line is you cannot change your genes but there are diet and lifestyle modifications you can make to play your hand the best you can. Exercise might be super important for some, or cold-water exposure, while for others eating ginger, curcumin (the active ingredient in turmeric), chilli peppers, garlic, and ginger will also be your friends.

But, like all the other discussions in this book, it's part of the jigsaw. You cannot hope to *just* do a DNA test in the hope that everything will turn out rosy. This is fine tuning.

Is your body on fire?

In the same way, inflammation is interesting but it's not the single thing that will make a huge difference to your energy, weight, mood or menopause symptoms.

Inflammation is at the root – or at least a major contributor – to the progression of practically every disease you can name and it ramps up a few notches in midlife. Your gut environment (the microbiome) is right at the centre of that. If you don't break foods down correctly, this can lead to harmful fermentation products getting into your bloodstream, heading to the liver where they can switch on inflammatory processes that result in your body storing more fat.

Food sensitivities (we're talking food intolerance rather than a true allergy) produce antibodies to 'problem foods' and these may vary from person to person. These IgG antibodies create low-level inflammation through the body and a huge variety of unwelcome symptoms. Signs of food intolerance vary greatly from one person to the next but some of them include weight that won't shift, bloating, headaches or migraines, runny nose, itchy or overly waxy ears, IBS, hives, fatigue, asthma, eczema, arthritis, blocked nose, or frequent ear infections.

If any of the symptoms of food intolerance seem to fit with how you are feeling, a fingerpick food intolerance test might yield some valuable insights but, to be very honest with you, if you are struggling to lose weight or your menopausal symptoms are out of control, you are probably looking in the wrong place.

I cannot tell you how many people get in touch asking about food intolerance testing. The reality is, I request very few because there is almost always a lot of work to be done elsewhere before the thought of food intolerance crosses my mind. By the time my clients have worked on my agenda and start seeing the results they've been looking for, it's never spoken of again. Not always, but often, food intolerance testing is the sign you're hunting for a magic pill.

> **10-second recap**
> Although many women assume something must be wrong with them if they can't lose weight, much of the time it's simply that what their body needs to work well has changed now they're in their 40s or 50s. However, there are some challenges that can put the brakes on weight loss and some become more likely in midlife: thyroid dysfunction, gut imbalance, and unhelpful genes (note: these don't change over time but diet and lifestyle do influence how they are expressed). All of these factors can be tested in my nutrition clinic.

PART TWO

CHAPTER 6
METABOLISM BOOSTING GUIDELINES

This part of the book is about food. It's the actual doing part and this may take a little time to get your head around, largely because, instead of doing whatever your usual thing is, I'm going to ask you to take another look at how your meals are made up and I'll give you some simple rules to follow as much as you can. Try your best. You don't have to do it all in a day.

You might choose to switch up some ingredients on your plate, take on a whole meal or jump in to fix all your meals at once. It's not a race. Everyone has a pace they like to do things. Keep in mind, this is not another diet you start on a Monday and it goes on for however long you can keep doing it until you can stand it no longer. If you want to start small, feel comfortable doing that until you take the leap into fixing the next meal, that's fine. This is about finding a system that works for you.

How you start the day matters - and here's why

Breakfast is the most important meal of the day and potentially the most dangerous. If you're into the type of fasting called intermittent fasting (spoiler alert, I think it's a good idea but with some specific modifications for midlife health), read 'breakfast' simply as the first meal of the day.

How you fuel yourself at the start of your daily eating journey really matters. You have an opportunity to do great things. In theory at least, your blood sugar levels should be nice and low. You're ready for food but you're not experiencing cravings. It's a *Sliding Doors* moment (remember that film?): a day with two futures and here's how it might play out.

You choose a savoury breakfast like an omelette or similar. Maybe you're feeling fruity and you go for a bowl of Greek yoghurt, some berries and topped with some chopped nuts and seeds. Neither take long to throw together and, whichever you choose, you're on your way pretty quickly.

Or you pour yourself a bowl of cereal, or maybe you just head straight out of the door and grab a croissant and a latte on the way into work.

In that first future, you're probably not hungry till lunch or certainly not ravenous. If you have a similarly balanced lunch (let's say for argument, soup and a chicken salad), you can power yourself right through the afternoon without incident - you're certainly not tempted by the Devon fudge Sandra brought back from holiday and can take or leave the doughnuts that arrived by way of celebrating someone's birthday. Unless you're going to be late home and need a snack, the evening meal is pretty straightforward, too. You're certainly not forced to eat your body weight in cheese as you hunt for something to cook.

Here's what that other future might look like:

A bowl of pretty much any cereal, marmite on toast or a croissant and latte. I didn't have time, okay?

Recriminations. What is wrong with me? I meant to start properly today. Going to be good for the rest of the day.

Mid-morning. Starving. Ooh, biscuits.

More recriminations. Never mind, I can get this back.

Is it lunch yet? I know I should have a salad, but I'm really busy. Leaves, quinoa. Don't have time for stuff with a fork. Just a sandwich and crisps. I won't have chocolate. Phew, that could have been a whole lot worse. This is definitely the last day I do this.

Fancy biscuits in a meeting are the best, and Sandra would feel offended if I didn't at least try her fudge. Tomorrow is the day I am officially getting back on this. Just one, okay, I'll take a second for later. Thank you.

Back home. Why am I so hungry today? Hunt through cupboards. Ugh. Nothing looks even slightly appealing. Pie and chips in the air fryer with cheese and biscuits while I wait? Today was a total disaster. Or maybe we should get a takeaway and I'll start over tomorrow? I'll get up in time for breakfast and make my own lunch. Tomorrow I will be a planning goddess.

Ooh, that thing's on TV. Don't want to miss that. And I deserve a little something after such a long day. Double decker, anyone?

Bed.

I don't say that to be critical. We're all busy but free-wheeling through life doesn't really work when it comes to feeding yourself or your family - and there are few things worse than a chorus of 'what's for dinner' when you get in the door and your answer is 'if you can find it, you can have it. Let the foraging begin.' I won't lie, the latter has happened way too often in my own home.

When you don't start the day with a meal that balances your blood sugar levels, the rest of the day will be an uphill struggle. Just like the smoker who has stubbed out her last cigarette, if you start the day with your sugars spiking, the cravings will follow you around like a lost pet for the remainder of the day and it will be hard to get back on track. You'll feel hungrier, have less energy, be more grumpy, and feel powerless when it comes to food temptations. You'll also have to deal with your disappointment with *yourself* (and that's always the worst). To top it all, the blood sugar rollercoaster you are on will probably result in you waking up in the middle of the night and maybe you'll get back to sleep and maybe you won't.

This is not an exaggeration. It's a very real possibility and I know that we have both been there and it's not pretty. In your twenties and thirties, your body was more forgiving, but things are different now and it's just the way it is.

I'm going to assume you want to fix this so you can just get back to feeling normal - as a minimum - if not great again. This is what we're doing in this chapter and, in fact, the rest of the book.

Let's pull in some of what we learned earlier...

In midlife, your body will typically be able to handle starchy carbs like potatoes, rice, pasta bread and sugar less well than before, so you'll need to watch how much of these things you eat and - importantly - you don't want to eat them on their own.

They empty glucose into the bloodstream quickly, causing a cascade of unfortunate events as I described earlier. It's not that any of that is wrong, per se. There will be days when you do have the fudge or the doughnut, just not all the time.

How can I stop my blood glucose spiking?

Make sure you always include in your meal things that will slow down how quickly the glucose lands in your bloodstream (protein, fat and fibre). Improve the quality of your food (opting for wholegrain foods over white or processed) and change the quantities of different types of food if you need to. Here's a guide.

- Always have a palm-sized amount of protein with every meal and snack.
- Fill the majority of your plate with veggies and salad (fibre).
- Go easy on the starchy carbs (bread, pastry, rice, pasta, and so on) and things containing added sugar (and never eat them on their own).
- Add a tablespoon of healthy fats to each meal.

I find it helps to have a little knowledge of some of the terms people use for food constituents - if only so you can keep up to speed with conversations about food you hear outside of this book. So, it helps to know what macros and micros are so you can nod or shake your head or have a view if you so wish.

I'm not usually one in my private consultations asking clients to 'track their macros'. That's usually the prevail of the gym bunnies, coached by personal trainers on their food, and who make multiple portions of the same meal and stash it in those takeaway containers in the fridge so they can have a chicken dinner six times a day. I'm not saying don't do that and the advice is wrong. It's just not my style, either as a practitioner or how I personally want to live my life. I'm all up for making multiple portions of a stew or a curry to keep in the freezer but I would cry if I opened up my fridge to find a day's worth of meals boxed up in front of me.

Macros and micros

Macros - the powerhouse trio of proteins, carbohydrates, and fats - are the backbone of your diet. Micros are the guardians of your wellbeing, and include the vitamins, minerals, and plant chemicals you need in smaller amounts to keep your body ticking along like a well-oiled machine.

What is protein?

'Protein' comes from the Greek word 'proteos', meaning primary or 'taking first place'. (That's one for quiz night). Protein gives you the building blocks of life and is found in muscle, bone, skin, hair, and virtually every other body part or tissue.

It's an oversimplification to say protein is what grows muscle, but it's certainly what you'll see people double up on when they no longer want to lose weight and want to sculpt and grow muscle. The reason body-builders love it so much is when they do heavy work, they create tiny tears in their muscles. Protein swoops in like a superhero to repair and rebuild the muscle fibres - just so you know, this is important for regular folk for things like wound healing. But proteins also make up the enzymes that power many chemical reactions, they make hormones and neurotransmitters - among other things - and can be a source of energy.

Proteins are important nutritionally because of the amino acids they contain. Animal sources of protein deliver all the amino acids you need (and we need a full spectrum to have the best health). Plant-based sources (soy, grains, legumes, nuts and seeds) do not always contain the full range of amino acids, so you need to eat a variety of the day to get all of the essential amino acids into your diet. 'Novel proteins' like textured vegetable protein (derived from soy) and Quorn (mycoprotein derived from fungus) are manufactured and have the same issues as other processed foods - they're just not that healthy for you whatever the marketing campaign behind them.

When it comes to your metabolism, here are some important things to know:
- Protein helps keep you feeling fuller for longer, much more so than carbs. It will also guard against a blood sugar spike, so you should always have protein with every meal and snack (if you're having one).
- Protein guards against muscle loss (we'll see in the next part of the book that this is super important).

- Of all the macros, protein taxes your body more to break it down, meaning it uses more energy/ calories to do the work aka it has the highest thermal effect of food (TEF).

How much protein?

This is the part where I say 'be sensible'. The World Health Organization (WHO) says a woman needs 0.75g of protein per kilo of her body weight with an upper limit of 1.5 kg per day. This is 45g to 90g per day for an 'average' woman weighing 60 kg (about 9 stone 6 or 132 pounds) with a sedentary lifestyle. The bodybuilding industry would tell you to triple it, which would be on the heavy side in my view. Although we can start getting the calculators out, I suggest you don't. When I'm working with clients I find that too much measuring of any kind takes up too much headspace when you just want to make your lunch, so let's move away from the numbers very quickly.

The palm of your hand is a decent enough measure for most people. For animal protein (meat, fish or seafood of any kind), go for one palm-size and thickness of protein at each meal or 2 or 3 eggs. For plant-based protein (tofu, tempeh, quorn, lentils, beans, etc), go for 1.5 palm size and thickness - no scales, just use your imagination. You can mix up your proteins. One of my favourite salads contains chicken, chickpeas, and pumpkin seeds.

What is fat and is it bad?

Healthy fats are found in oily fish like salmon, trout, mackerel and sardines, nuts, seeds of all kinds, olives and olive oil, and avocados. You want them in the most natural state possible, which is why highly processed oils for cooking are a bad idea (like vegetable and sunflower oil) but that's a story for another day.

Fat has a bad rap thanks to years of terrible science incorrectly signposting fat as the main cause of obesity and heart disease. We now know it's the refined carbs and sugars that are to blame but Big Food (and other vested interests) are still encouraging people to eat very low-fat diets. This is not the answer to fixing your metabolism because the amount of fat you are eating is very unlikely to be at the root of your problems. Here are some other important things to know about fat for that pub quiz:

- Fat is also important for protecting your organs, maintaining normal body temperature, and regulating inflammation, mood and nerve function.
- Every cell membrane in your body is made of fat – the brain is 60% fat.
- Many hormones are made from fat. These are known as steroid hormones and they govern stress, sex, and immune function. Oestrogen, progesterone and testosterone are steroid hormones.
- Diets high in starchy carbohydrates and sugar turn on the fat production factory in your liver (lipogenesis), and this causes high cholesterol and high triacylglycerols while lowering good (HDL) cholesterol.
- Omega 3 fats (from oily fish, walnuts, chia and flax seeds) are very anti-inflammatory and great for supporting hormone production and mood.

What are carbohydrates?

No food is inherently bad (or good, for that matter). Many serial dieters might fear carbs and, while it's true there are no essential carbohydrates in the same way there are essential proteins (essential amino acids) and essential fats (essential fatty acids like omegas 3 and 6), they still fulfil an important role in the body since carbohydrates are effectively everything else I haven't mentioned above, from fruit and veggies to legumes and wholegrains.

In incredibly simplistic terms, we can roughly categorise carbs as being fibre (fruit and veg), starch (bread, pasta, rice) and sugar (sugary treats, pastries and cakes and so on).

The carbs we want more of are those that contain plenty of fibre as fibre slows down how quickly starches and glucose enter the bloodstream.

The food you actually eat is mostly a combination of these different macronutrients. Apart from sucrose, which is 100% carbohydrate and oils, which are in themselves 100% fat, other foods will have elements of something else. Though I'm categorising meat, fish, and eggs as protein, the reality is, they contain both protein and fat in the same way dairy does. It's a similar situation with fruit and veg, and grains, beans and pulses, which contain both carbs and protein at the same time. Nuts, seeds and avocados contain all three macros.

What to eat

The next chapter deals with exactly what to eat and will give you some practical guidance that makes all the stuff above (and, for that matter, the earlier part of the book) make sense. What I can tell you is this book is based on the real science of what midlife women should eat more of the time than not. I'm not talking about birthdays, Christmas and holiday holidays, religious or otherwise. Those days, we need different agreements with ourselves about what we want to eat because they are special. I just want to acknowledge here that there are days at specific points in your cycle when you want to eat what you want to eat and you should listen to your body - within reason.

Your menstrual cycle & what you feel like eating

If you are in perimenopause and still cycling (you are still having a period even if it's become a bit intermittent), this bit is for you…

Once you fix your diet so you're no longer on that blood sugar rollercoaster of cravings, hunger and recriminations (by eating protein and trimming out many of the unnecessary carbs, which we'll talk about in the next chapter), you will feel great but there may still be times that you feel you need more stodge, and that's often the week before your period. That's due to the interplay between your lady hormones, the fat-storage hormone insulin and the stress hormone cortisol.

Early in your cycle, when oestrogen is high (it's all relative), insulin trends lower. For the first couple of weeks of your cycle when oestrogen is on the up, you will find eating well easy and get more satisfaction from lighter, more balanced meals. The hormonal mix at this stage of your cycle makes you feel brighter and more positive. You'll be more patient, more energetic, sociable, focused, curious and more creative.

I'm basing this narrative on a 28-day cycle, which is for illustrative purposes only. A very small proportion of women will have a cycle that is exactly 28 days.

In perimenopause, you might find some cycles are shorter and lighter, while others are longer and you wake up to a scene looking like you've been killed in your bed.

As you get to week four - the run-up to your cycle when the body is making progesterone - you are more sensitive to the effects of the stress hormone cortisol and you lose your sensitivity to insulin. This makes fasting (if you're a fan of this practice - and more on this in chapters nine and ten) much harder and you crave starchy food. That's the time to lean into warming foods and make friends with sweet potatoes and other root vegetables, enjoy dark chocolate, and take more care of your self-care rather than get heavily involved in the cake aisle at the supermarket, whatever you think your body might be telling you. As an aside, if you make the changes I suggest in the book, I promise that this time of the month won't nearly be as difficult as you have felt it before.

10-second recap

Eating protein at every meal is key as it slows down how quickly glucose lands in your bloodstream. Make sure you start the day right with a protein-packed breakfast. Fibre from veggies also helps and will keep you feeling full. Fat is not bad for you and omega-3 fats (found in oily fish, walnuts, chia and flaxseeds) help lower inflammation. No food is banned (that's the fastest way to make a gal break a 'diet') but lots of starchy foods are not your friend in perimenopause and beyond.

CHAPTER 7
EXACTLY WHAT TO EAT

The easiest and the best advice I can give you to begin with is to eat real food. Avoid the processed stuff we kid ourselves it's OK to eat (and are tempted to do that most of the time). I see people massively over-complicate eating by trying to follow all the rules of all the different possible diets. Hopefully this chapter will help simplify things so that you haven't got so much information flying around in your head when it comes to choosing what you'll eat - and, of course, so that you can get your metabolism back on track, rev up your energy levels, kill your cravings and experience a better menopause.

This is what I mean by real v processed:

Real food is meat and fish that is whole or chopped, from the butcher, fishmonger or the fresh aisle in the supermarket. It could be salted/ cured meat or fish like smoked salmon or plain cured bacon. It's also tofu and tempeh, lentils, beans, and chickpeas. Milk, butter, yoghurt (natural or authentic Greek yoghurt, not Greek-style yoghurt and definitely not 0% fat yoghurt), and cheese. Fruit and vegetables in their whole or chopped/ diced/ shredded state and fruit - not juice, which has almost all of the fibre squeezed out. The best for your blood sugars are cold climate fruits like berries and cherries, apples, pears, plums, in case you're wondering, since they naturally contain less sugar. Nuts and seeds and unsweetened butters made from them. Wholegrain brown rice, brown rice pasta, quinoa, oats. Water, tea and coffee, and herbal teas.

Processed food is deli-style cured meat/ sliced meat in packages, tinned meat (though tinned fish is OK), meat or fish in breadcrumbs, batter and with any marinade you have not made yourself as this is usually very high in sugar.

Pre-prepped veggie side dishes like pre-made cauliflower cheese, creamed spinach, breaded mushrooms and the like. Cans and cartons of drink, fruit juice. Anything else with added sugar of any kind, including treacle, agave and honey (yes, I know honey is, strictly speaking, natural but I'm including it here since it will mess up your blood sugar levels). White pasta and rice, pastries, breakfast cereals, pies and pastries, cakes and biscuits, dried fruit, jars and packets of sauces, fruity yoghurts.

Most condiments like ketchup, sweet chilli and flavoured mayo. Jams, jellies and most toast toppings.

These days, this junk even has its own term: Ultra Processed Foods. If it includes a list of ingredients as long as your arm and you don't recognise some of the stuff you see, welcome to the world of UPFs.

I'm not asking you to suddenly change everything you do, or saying that all will be lost over a spoon of chocolate spread or a couple of squirts of tommy K. I want to be clear with you about the things that will be best for your midlife metabolism. The goal of my book and, in fact, my whole nutrition ethos is *metabolic flexibility*, which is training your body to work better so you can have high days and holidays on the food front (but probably not as often as you have been) without gaining weight or feeling low in energy.

Yes, it is a little mysterious and vague to talk about 'balance' but do your best to eat real food most of the time. Don't get too worked up about a jar of ready-made sauce on the busiest weeknight, especially if it stops you phoning for a takeaway or hitting the f**k-it button.

You can start with one meal, or you go pretty much all in. There's no hurry and this isn't a race. Just do what feels right.

Start by ditching sugar

One of the easiest initial steps is to cut out added sugar. It's not the only step I want you to take but it's such a foundational piece, I created a mini course to help you easily and painlessly do exactly that, and it's called the Midlife Sugar Detox.

The beauty of this programme is it helps you figure out how to fill the large hole in your diet that sugar might leave.

Sugar is fattening because it forces your body to make more insulin both in the short and long term. It raises blood glucose and insulin is immediately made, and it encourages insulin resistance, which means the body makes more and more insulin over time.

Sugar is pretty much the only thing you can eat that has zero nutritional value. Some processed foods are going on for 100% sugar - like sweets, which are nothing more than coloured, flavoured sugar. The treat-sized bag of very famous squishy hearts and fried eggs has only 85 calories but there is nothing to offset the four different types of sugar (without counting the very concentrated fruit juices, which are used as intense sweeteners) that will inevitably spike your blood glucose.

Of course, you can look at a packet of sweets like these or a muffin and you know it will contain sugar. Big Food knows you might already be aware sugar is a 'bad thing' and they're terrified you're going to figure out just how bad so they like to list sugar in all kinds of cunning ways on food labels to deceive you so you'll need your wits about you to outsmart them.

There are scores of different names for sugar and many of them you won't have heard of before. All exert a similar effect on your blood glucose levels. Since you might be on the look-out for sugar and not like that it sits right at the top of the ingredients list, you'll likely see it featured under a few different names, all listed individually. Do not be fooled. That little treat bag of sweets I mentioned earlier contains glucose syrup (that's sugar syrup by the way), sugar (not syrup but otherwise identical), dextrose (anything with 'ose' at the end is a sugar), and caramelised sugar syrup plus the concentrated fruit juice.

Sugar has a lot of aliases

To fool you further, you might find products labelled sugar-free where in fact they contain one or more other ingredients that are natural sweeteners but the effect on your blood sugar remains the same. These include concentrated grape juice (often used in snacks for toddlers), honey and agave nectar. Ideally, ditch these from your diet too.

My advice is, become a label checking ninja. This sounds exhausting but you're probably buying the same foods over and over (it's not like you're shopping for a different mayonnaise each time you go to the supermarket), so it's worth taking a little time to research the best condiments that are lowest in sugar once and then it's done. By research, I mean stand in the supermarket aisle or look at the ingredients in the detailed description if you're shopping online.

What you'll almost certainly find is that the vast majority of condiments are full of sugar. The worst offenders are ketchup, brown and barbecue sauce, sweet chilli sauce, relish, honey mustard, salad dressings, Teriyaki and other marinades/ dipping sauces. In case you're wondering, the best shop-bought options are pesto, tahini, and regular mustard.

What to eat for breakfast

People talk about breakfast being the most important meal of the day and it is but maybe not for the reason you think. When you have a decent breakfast (I'll explain what that looks like in a moment), you are less likely to snack on things that your metabolism won't like.

A protein-rich breakfast is the order of the day. This will keep you feeling full till lunch and will stop your cravings. My clients almost can't believe the difference this makes. If you make the best choices at breakfast, it sets you up for the day. If you choose croissants and anything else that upsets your glucose levels, you will be chasing your cravings all day and will almost certainly feel like crashing at your desk midway through the afternoon.

There's no need to come up with 20 go-to breakfasts. Aim to pin down three that you love. You'll need a couple for during the week and a weekend option that could be more elaborate if you fancy it.

Authentic Greek yoghurt, cherries/ berries (frozen are fine), a tablespoon of chopped nuts or seeds (flaxseeds have added benefits for perimenopausal women, which I discuss in Chapter 8 - Foods that help with weight loss).

Authentic Greek yoghurt, berries and 2 tbsp no sugar granola - either make some yourself or invest some time Googling or checking the back of packets in the supermarket. You'll want one with no sugar and the like and maybe a smidge of maple syrup. It might even be called 'low carb' or 'keto'. Really, it's just bringing a tiny bit of crunch. It's not the main deal.

Scrambled egg (2-3 eggs) - jazz it up with herbs, pesto, add some smoked salmon.

2-3 egg omelette with whatever you have in your fridge. Even a plain one with chopped fresh herbs can be lovely. Serve with some wilted spinach (sounds fancy, but you can just heat it in a dry frying pan or use a dash of real olive oil and not one of those nasty pretend sprays) and some chopped avocado.

Breakfast traybake - 2 slices of nitrate/ sugar free bacon or 2 slices halloumi or 2 chicken/veggie sausages with plum tomatoes, Portobello mushroom and a handful of cherry tomatoes baked in the oven.

Huevos Rancheros or Shakshuka - lovely weekend breakfasts - topped with avocado, a squeeze of lime if you're feeling fancy and some chopped coriander. Takes longer to make but is well worth the effort.

Protein pancakes made with oats or ground almonds (there are all kinds of recipes on the internet including those made with more egg than regular pancakes, or cottage cheese) - try them with Greek yoghurt and berries.

Porridge (4 tbsp oats) made with unsweetened almond milk, handful of berries, 1 tbsp flaxseeds, and a drizzle of unsweetened almond butter. For many midlife women, porridge can be too starchy, so see how you go. I recommend adding a scoop of vanilla or chocolate protein powder to give the meal more substance and keep you feeling fuller. Purists would argue protein powder is processed, while this is true, real life for many of us is not 100% perfect. The goal of this book is not to turn you into a nutritional gnome or clean-eating purist but to help you find your own magic formula that works with your actual life.

What to eat for lunch

Lunch definitely needs some planning, in fact all your meals do if you don't want to end up in that familiar territory of the sandwich and crisps or takeaway pasta salad, neither of which are helpful for your midlife metabolism.

Salad.

There are a couple of big barriers when it comes to making salads. One of them is that people often can't think of what to put in a salad without it being painfully boring. Here, I'm thinking of the ham, cheese, tomato and radish salads my Grandma used to force upon me. A salad is a celebration of seasonal loveliness.

The other potential pitfall is you find the dream salad, you throw absolutely everything you love into it, and you eat it every day. It doesn't matter how amazing it is, pretty soon you're going to get sick of it. So then it's 'salads don't work for me' and you're back in the less healthy world of the sandwich.

You'll definitely want to have a couple of salad variations pinned down. Take your cue from those big lunch outlets. Do they put every possible ingredient into a single salad? Of course not. Instead, they find tasty combinations of a handful of ingredients, giving them variously an Italian, Spanish, Japanese, French or Greek spin, for example. So maybe create an Italian-themed one involving protein like chicken, olives, artichokes, sun dried tomatoes along with red onion, cucumber and leaves. And a Mediterranean or Greek-themed one with falafel/ hummus or feta and olives. Think of a few 'set recipes' you could do so your lunch-making is more 'I'm having the Italian one' rather than throwing everything you can find in the fridge into your lunchbox.

Use this simple formula to make your own:

1. Pick the leaves. Romaine lettuce, lambs lettuce, baby gem, oak leaf, endive, spinach, chicory, radicchio, rocket, watercress, red cabbage, bagged leaf mix.

    Note: iceberg lettuce contains virtually no nutrients and it is possibly the dullest and most tasteless of your options. Rotate your greens, have different ones every day/week. This is one of the easiest ways to bring in more food variety.

    Add unlimited non-starchy veg (but remember the rule employed by the professional pre-made salad makers on switching up the variety). This includes **Raw** red onions, spring onions, cucumber, tomatoes, avocados (½ max), peppers, celery. **Roasted** asparagus, red onions, peppers, courgettes, aubergines. **Steamed** asparagus (or roasted), broccoli, cauliflower, green beans - all cooked, then cooled. One portion

(fist size) of starchy veg (optional) **Raw** carrots (grated). **Roasted** sweet potato, squash/ pumpkin, beetroot, butternut squash. Or cooked quinoa (obviously not a veg but it comes into this section nonetheless).
2. Protein (palm-sized total, unless detailed below, palm-and-a-half for veggie sources - combine proteins if you like). Choose from the following: **cooked poultry/meat** chicken, turkey, beef, pork, lamb. **Fish** tuna (tinned or steak), salmon (tinned, smoked, fillet), trout, prawns. **Cheese (30 g):** mature cheddar (grated), Roquefort (crumbled), feta (crumbled), goat's cheese, parmesan shavings, halloumi (grilled, baked). **Pulses (tinned)** kidney beans, butter beans, cannellini beans, flageolet beans, chickpeas, lentils (pouch/tinned). **Nuts** walnuts, pecans, pine nuts, hazelnuts, cashews, flaked almonds. **Other** eggs (boiled), tofu.
3. Add a garnish. One tablespoon (optional) **jarred antipasto** like sun dried tomatoes, roasted peppers, olives, jalapeños, artichokes. **Seeds** like sunflower seeds, pumpkin seeds, sesame seeds. **Herbs** parsley, basil, coriander. **Dressings** 2 tbsp extra virgin olive oil, 1 tbsp vinegar, 1 tsp mustard, salt, pepper. OR 2 tbsp extra virgin olive oil, 1 tbsp lemon juice, salt, pepper.

Winters can feel trickier. People often feel like ditching the salad days once the threat of having to get into your swimsuit or skimpy summer clothes has gone and there is often the feeling you need more carbs (don't skip the starchy veg, above). You probably, in fact, need more *hot* food.

Soup.
Maybe the office canteen has something decent, maybe one of those lunchy places does. Failing that, you can get some pretty decent hot food flasks so you can bring your own. Soup and salad works if you need something more substantial for lunch. You can eat it in one sitting, or you can have the soup as a snack and eat the salad later (or whichever way round, really it doesn't matter).

For soup, choose any protein-based soup but avoid those containing potatoes, rice or pasta and hold the croutons. Wondering what to put with it? Two rough oatcakes spread with hummus, a thin slice of rye bread (try it, you might surprise yourself) or - and I haven't had a client yet who hasn't loved these - my low carb cheese scones (see the recipe and try for yourself at https://www.foodfabulous.co.uk/post/cheese-scone).

Left-overs from last night's dinner also work, especially if you're working from home or have the facility to heat it up properly in the office kitchen.

What to eat for your evening meal

There are almost a gazillion different options for main meals, possibly more, I haven't counted. Really, you're looking to create a plate that looks like this:

- Protein (about palm sized or 1.5 the size if you're doing veggie protein - don't overthink it)
- Lots of veggies and/or salad
- A little healthy fat
- Easy on the starches like potatoes, rice, bread and pasta. Instead, lean into quinoa (you'll need to flavour it as it tastes of nothing at all) and 'faux carbs' like cauliflower rice.

The overall goal is to have your whole diet be less carb-heavy so that your body very quickly runs down the glucose in the blood and the stored glucose and has to go find the fat stored on your body to use that as energy. That does not mean do not have *any* carbs, but at your evening meal we want to really squeeze these low. This will become easier the more balanced your blood sugar levels are. At the same time as squeezing the carbs a little, you should add in more salady veg or vegetables to fill you up and are also excellent for health in general.

I think it's a mistake to outlaw any food because this inevitably leads to feelings of restriction but we do have to work with the science and that tells us midlife women can usually tolerate fewer starchy foods due to their changing metabolism.

I want this to be a book that is approachable for all women and not women who want to get hardcore about their diet. You learnt in previous chapters that, when you're in midlife, having a lot of starchy carbs doesn't really work with your metabolism. And yet there are times that you will want your starchy carbs and that's that. So I'm going to give you some very specific guidance on this so you don't end up starting well and then suddenly the evening meal becomes a bowl of pasta and low-fat sauce again.

More guiding principles

For more meals than not, stick to the golden rules of blood sugar balance. Eat a varied, colourful diet and do the stuff you know to do.

In the run up to your period, hormonal changes might make you feel hungrier and crave more starchy foods so bring in a little more of these but go for the good ones. If you need a wrap at lunchtime, make it a wholemeal wrap or protein wrap, and fill it with protein and leaves. If you need a little starch for your evening meal (and try not to do this every day), add some - sweet potatoes do the job really well as does quinoa. I want this to be a life change, not a diet you suffer for as long as you need to before you can stop doing it and get back to what wasn't working before. It wasn't working for a reason. I'll give you some upper limit guidelines in a moment. Once you have rebalanced your blood sugar levels, you will be able to read what your body is actually telling you. If you've not yet done that work, the messages will be confusing.

Do not double carb, by which I mean if there is a roast dinner, choose what matters most – Yorkshire pudding or a roast potato – and, in the example of a pie made with either potato or pastry, do not have any starchy sides like mashed potato, chips, rice or pasta on the side.

As we've discussed, the vast majority of the foods we eat cause the body to make some kind of hormonal response. There is a huge scale with things like broccoli and leafy green veg at one end of the spectrum and potatoes at the other end. And even for potatoes, there is a sliding scale where chips/fries have a greater impact on blood sugar levels than new potatoes, allowing you to eat more of those things that contain the least 'sugars'.

See the list below to give you a good idea of appropriate portion size of various foods. You will see that basmati rice gets you more bang for your buck compared to long grain rice, and so on.

** One important thing to note is this: when you first make changes to your diet your body may play tricks on you to let you know that something has changed. Your body isn't really a fan of change, it just wants to stay the same (that's homeostasis, which you might remember from biology class at school). The signals your body might give could be that you feel hungry, or you get a headache for a few days or you feel a bit more fatigued than normal. There is really nothing wrong, but your body wants to let you know that something is different and it is not sure about it. This will change.**

Upper limits on starchy foods

Since foods that release their sugars into the bloodstream quickly cause the body to make more insulin (the fat storage hormone), I advise keeping an eye on how much you eat in one meal. You can see how you get more quantity for the same impact on your blood glucose when you choose wholegrain varieties over white varieties, and (for potatoes) a specific way of cooking.

The following relates to the cooked product:
- Carrot 160g (about 1 large)
- Beetroot 110g (about 1 large)
- Quinoa 65g (about 2 handfuls)
- Cous cous 25g (about 1 handful)
- Regular white pasta 35g (one small handful)
- Wholewheat pasta 40g (about 1 handful)
- Brown rice or basmati 40g (about 1 handful)
- Long grain rice 25g (2 tbsp)
- Corn on the cob 60g (half a cob)
- Baked potato/ mash 60g (half a potato)
- New potato 75g (approx 3)
- French fries 3

What, no recipes?

Dust off the books you already own!

I'm deliberately not including recipes as part of this book (but skip to the resources section if you really cannot do without). I'm betting you have more than enough perfectly good books in your kitchen already. When you have an hour or so, take some sticky notes, grab a couple of books and start to flag those recipes that fit the bill. There are some recipe books I use a great deal and amend specific recipes. I will omit the drizzle of honey over satay chicken because I don't think it adds much to the dish, for example. I might change the suggested side dishes or accompaniments. If worse comes to worst, I can serve with some steamed broccoli or a big salad. Don't overthink this exercise.

There are also probably some meals you are already eating that you can tweak, and this is the easiest thing to do. Customise what you already know. Here are some ideas and how you can make them midlife metabolism friendly.

- Chicken and vegetable tray bake - go easy on the potatoes
- Steak (don't worry about the sauce) with a generous salad - add wedges made from ½ a sweet potato if you fancy
- Tagine with cauliflower rice or quinoa rather than rice
- Chilli (veggie or meat) with cauliflower rice or quinoa rather than rice
- Bolognese or lentil ragu with courgetti or a mix of pasta and veg
- Curry served with cauliflower rice or quinoa instead of regular rice
- Grilled or baked fish or chicken with your own marinade (I love the flavours of rosemary, lemon and garlic or Thai vibes with garlic, ginger, chilli and fresh coriander and these work equally well on chicken or firm tofu) with loads of veggies
- Oven baked white fish on a bed of lentils

Should I be snacking?

Ideally not, but it depends. Why so wishy-washy?

Advice changes over time and you might have heard people talking about eating little and often or grazing. My advice? Don't. You learnt at the beginning of the book that blood sugar and insulin spikes are bad for your health and terrible news for your menopause. Part of the problem with how the human body consumes food and uses energy these days is that most people eat the 'wrong' things (too much sugar, too many refined carbs) and too often, causing the body to repeatedly send in the fat storage hormone insulin. You can probably sense that this is not a good thing. Your body needs periods of rest, too. And your digestive system needs rest. The ideal scenario is to have a decent blood sugar balancing meal at breakfast, wait until your lunch, and then leave a gap before you have your evening meal, with a nice long break from eating overnight.

Your body does not need this continuous onslaught of food all day long.

It's normal to feel hungry between meals. In fact, it's how it should be. This is different from that ravenous, starving-your-face-off feeling that comes from your blood sugar levels being out of whack, or underfeeding.

Oftentimes people eat for reasons that have nothing to do with actual hunger - I mentioned Sandra's Devon shareables earlier and everyone's instinct to dive in. Then there's habit, and then boredom. If you're not hungry, don't snack. If you fancy a snack, just check in with yourself and ask, 'Am I really hungry?'

A further reason for that snacky feeling is you haven't had a decent protein-packed breakfast. If you already had a low-protein breakfast, don't worry about it today but try to include more protein tomorrow.

Let's be real, sometimes the gap between one meal and the next can get stretched, especially if you're caught late at work or you're out and about. And it's worth noting, one thing that comes up in all the research on snacking is that there is no official definition of what a 'snack' actually is, making it impossible to know if people are eating too many meals or too many snacks.

Here's my view:

A meal is larger, a snack is *much* smaller and its job is to tide you over - and nothing more - until your next meal, especially if the gap between meals is over four hours. Not an official definition, but there you go. So, ideally you'll want to get out of the habit of snacking because, if you're not careful, you can eat a lot in those sneaky mini meals - English Apples & Pears (the fruit marketing board for these fruit, who knew?) interviewed 2,000 people in a survey on snacking back in 2019 and found that women were typically eating 1,200 calories a day outside of their regular meals, nearly two thirds of their expected calorie allowance.

If you need ideas for snacks, try these:
- Hummus and crudités (like red pepper, cucumber, celery and carrot sticks)
- Apple and a small portion of cheese (matchbox size - like the ones they sell in netted bags in the supermarket)

- Nuts - a small palmful
- Apple, pear, satsuma or 2 plums with a small palmful (about 5-10) of unsalted nuts
- Small pot natural yoghurt with a good handful of berries and 6-8 chopped nuts
- Cottage cheese boats - little gem lettuce 'boat' holding about 150g cottage cheese and top with chopped cucumber or other salad veg
- Cottage cheese with a handful of berries
- Miso soup
- 2 hard-boiled eggs with a handful of spinach (often available in supermarkets and lunchtime eateries if you can't be bothered to make your own)
- DIY trail mix - leave out the high-natural-sugar dried fruit. Make yours from a mix of nuts and seeds, including something exotic like cacao nibs for a real treat. Portion size is a handful
- Fresh coconut - filling, thanks to the fibre content, and contains healthy fats. The brave might buy their own coconut, but plenty of supermarkets and luncheries sell their own pre-packed pots. Snack size: 80g

10-second recap

Eat real food as much of the time as you can but don't lose the plot over the odd jar of sauce or ready meal. Ditching added sugar (including all of its aliases as well as agave and honey) is a good place to start. When you start the day with a protein-rich breakfast, you're less likely to experience cravings through the rest of the day.

CHAPTER 8
FOODS THAT HELP YOU LOSE WEIGHT

I feel bad for having a chapter with this title because I suspect I might have lured you here under false pretences. Here's the thing, unless you get the food strategy right (by this I mean balancing your blood sugar levels), you're wasting your time focussing on individual foods. The big picture is this: balance your blood sugar levels, sleep, take care of your stress and your happiness, and build muscle. The rest are the fine details that, on their own, will have little impact. I'm sorry to be the one to break it to you, but those downloadable guides you see on social media that promise doing this 'one trick' as the solution to your weight loss woes are utter bullshit.

There are millions of internet pages dedicated to foods that help you burn fat but what it essentially boils down to is this: eat real food, eat lean protein, cut out treat foods, eat fermented foods and others that are good for the gut, eat healthy fats, eat dark chocolate. There, that should save you a bunch of hours. There are no shortcuts. And yet (she says mysteriously)...

Green tea

We have to start with green tea, which is probably the healthiest tea on the planet thanks largely to the polyphenols called epigallocatechin-3-gallate (ECCG). It's actually the same plant as the black tea you use to make your builder's tea but far less processed. It contains caffeine (though less than a cup of coffee) so that has fat-burning properties in and of itself, and it's chock full of antioxidants that fight free radicals that cause oxidative stress. If you've ever bought a face cream for the claims around it combatting the free radicals that cause lines and wrinkles, you'd likely be far better off (not to mention richer) with a box of green tea.

Green tea is anti-inflammatory, chemo-protective (offers some protection against cancer), antibacterial, antiviral, anti-arthritic and neuroprotective (protects the brain), and scientists are fascinated by its apparent ability to burn fat. The mechanisms are not entirely clear and the research is ongoing, but it seems to be beneficial for your metabolism by influencing the 'master metabolic switch' called AMPK (adenosine monophosphate-activated protein kinase, in case you're wondering), helping regulate appetite by telling your body you're full and upregulating some of the helpful genes in the fatburn pathway, and helping with insulin sensitivity.

Most of the studies have been done on green tea extract but that's not to say you cannot get this from the tea itself; you'll just need more of it. If you are not sipping it already, add it to your shopping list. (Side note: don't go hunting out high-strength green tea extracts since some people can't deal with that level of supplementation).

Practical takeaway: A cup or two a day is likely worth a try.

Coffee

Despite its reputation for being something to cut out of your diet, research over a long period of time has demonstrated coffee is a good thing overall and there are health benefits that range from longevity to protection against neurodegenerative conditions like Alzheimer's and Parkinson's. While it's true that coffee does have a small impact on blood pressure (so take care if your levels are raised), research shows that women who drank coffee had a reduced risk of heart disease. When it comes to weight loss, the winning ingredients seem to be the polyphenols and caffeine. Caffeine is found in almost every fat loss supplement because it's one of a very small number of substances proven to help with fat burning. Research shows that it can boost your metabolic rate by up to 13% depending on which study you read. If you combine it with exercise, it's even more powerful - coffee drunk an hour before exercise was found to have increased fat burning.

Since we are interested in all things blood glucose here and anything that might increase sensitivity to insulin while lowering the risk of developing type 2 diabetes is a good thing, there's more promising research about coffee. One large-scale study of over half a million people demonstrated the risk of developing type 2 diabetes or insulin resistance was 4% lower in coffee drinkers, and this might be to do with links to reducing inflammation. The link was strongest in habitual coffee drinkers who drank ground coffee, like espresso or filtered coffee, which boosts levels of the hormone adiponectin (important for managing glucose levels and breaking down fat) and the anti-inflammatory cytokines, while decreasing levels of the proinflammatory proteins. But the effect was only seen in non-smokers - so not everyone gets to benefit.

Practical takeaway: If you like a black coffee, this is good news. Enjoy a couple of good-quality coffees but do it in the morning so there is a lower risk of the caffeine disrupting your sleep hormones. Some people get jittery when they drink coffee. If this is you, don't start drinking coffee for the health benefits. And, if the only way you can drink coffee is with a litre of milk and sugar, the extra energy and sugars (even in the milk) are not worth the potential gain.

Ginger and chilli

These two beauts also activate that master metabolic switch AMPK through an effect on the ADIPOQ gene. There won't be a test, so don't worry about remembering the name. Just know these are good things to be cooking with.

Practical takeaway: Since no one really knows how much of these foods you'd need to eat to get the therapeutic benefits, use them where you can. If you're a fan of dishes from the Middle East, India or Far East, these will be familiar ingredients. Fill your boots.

Turmeric

Turmeric (specifically the active part curcumin) is helpful for all kinds of midlife woes and, though you can buy this little root both fresh and ground in supermarkets, the reality is that you'll probably need a supplement to get a therapeutic dose into your diet - though every little helps. Turmeric is well-known for its anti-inflammatory properties and it's often top of the list of supplements for people who have arthritis. There's some work that shows it can suppress fat tissue growth, reduce blood pressure and cholesterol. It also features in most supplements for metabolic health for its role in regulating blood glucose levels and improving insulin sensitivity.

Turmeric is also a phytoestrogen. We'll come on to that in a moment.

Practical takeaway: Turmeric can be used in a wide variety of dishes as a flavour enhancer (think curries, rice dishes and so on), with eggs, teas and turmeric latte, but it's hard to consume enough of it to see the benefits so consider supplementing too.

Rhubarb

Rhubarb is a good thing. It goes surprisingly well with another one of these beneficial ingredients - ginger. Rhubarb's power lies in its rheinic acid content. Remember the FATSO gene earlier in the book that dials up hunger and dials down satiety so you don't get the signal to stop eating? Rhubarb helps modulate that - in a good way, obviously. Let's not forget this vegetable (even though we eat it like a fruit) is also full of fibre which on another level is very beneficial for balancing blood glucose.

Obviously, if you're having it as a super sweet rhubarb crumble, you're negating the effect somewhat but everything has its place.

Practical takeaway: If you need your rhubarb to be sweet, there's nothing terrible about adding a touch of Stevia, which is a healthier sweetener than most of the other options. But don't knock unsweetened rhubarb - try it poached or stewed with a little vanilla pod and ginger and add it to authentic Greek or unsweetened coconut yoghurt.

Sirt foods

You may also have heard of Sirt foods. There was even a whole diet created around them. There is a family of proteins called sirtuins that influence gene expression and can impact cellular functions, including metabolism, stress response, longevity, and inflammation. One of the most well-studied is SIRT1, which influences how fat is stored and used in the body. This so-called 'skinny' gene gets activated by factors including caloric restriction (eating less than your body needs) and consuming bioactive compounds found in specific foods or that activate sirtuins ('sirt foods').

These are Sirt foods:
- Dark chocolate (at least 85% cocoa)
- Bird's eye chilli
- Kale
- Parsley
- Green tea
- Turmeric
- Olives and olive oil
- Rocket
- Medjool dates
- Capers
- Walnuts
- Onions
- Tofu
- Miso
- Apples
- Strawberries
- Citrus fruits
- Blueberries
- Red wine
- Coffee

Practical takeaway: In theory, this all makes sense. We know that foods are chemical messages in the body but, when it comes to hard and fast science, the research is patchy. Luckily, these are all healthful foods that I would recommend, so that's enough reason to get them into your diet. Eat a couple of portions a day if you can.

Would I eat a diet that only contained foods that upregulate the genes you want to tinker with? No and neither should you. We both have a life to live and, while 'functional foods' can be helpful, midlife is the time to embrace the overarching strategy rather than the minutiae of eating blueberries and walnuts. No one ever needs to take eating that far.

Cinnamon

Cinnamon is a popular culinary spice and, to be fair, all herbs and spices are a great thing to add to your diet, whether fresh, frozen or dried. As an aside, these all count in a bid to eat a more varied diet, and many of these ingredients have some kind of medicinal value. Don't believe me? Herbs, in particular, have been used by people from ancient times and the word 'drug' comes from the French word 'drogue', which means Dry Herb and reflects the origins of modern pharmacology from the study of humble medicinal plants. Aspirin, for example, came from willow bark and morphine from the opium poppy, but I digress. In olden times, if you weren't being treated with leeches, you were probably being medicated with herbs. Many are anti-inflammatory and we should use more of them for good health, particularly as it's easy to do so.

But back to cinnamon, which can be added to more dishes than you might imagine. It contains a host of vitamins and minerals as well as other helpful components like cinnamaldehyde, cinnamate and cinnamic acid, which give cinnamon anti-diabetic, anti-microbial, antioxidant, and anti-inflammatory properties. It helps improve sensitivity to insulin and there have been a multitude of studies of studies that draw links between cinnamon supplementation and a reduction in body fat.

Practical takeaway: 1-2 teaspoons of cinnamon powder or 1-inch cinnamon bark per day. Sprinkle on porridge, add to smoothies, use as a flavour enhancer for quinoa or rice, add to chilli, make a cinnamon and turmeric latte, add to apple sauce or home-made low carb granola, and bring an extra layer of flavour to Indian-inspired curries and Moroccan meatballs and tagines.

Phytoestrogens

These are naturally-occurring plant-based chemicals, which are structurally similar to oestrogen and exert a weak oestrogenic effect on your body. They're one of nature's genius ingredients called adaptogens. This means they can either replicate or counteract the effects of oestrogen. They either help out by giving where oestrogen might be lacking - like perimenopause and beyond - or they take, where there might be too much oestrogen as in conditions linked to oestrogen dominance (or unopposed oestrogen as we now call it) such as endometriosis, fibroids or PMT.

One of the many things we now know about women's experience of menopause is that women in the Far East typically experience fewer symptoms than women in the West. The reason? These women, thanks to culture and tradition, eat more of one of the particularly powerful phytoestrogens. While synthetic oestrogens (think HRT) have been linked to unfavourable outcomes like increased risk of some hormone-driven cancers, there are no known health risks from eating more plant foods like phytoestrogens. The absorption of phytoestrogens depends on a healthy gut, as there must be enough healthy bacteria to convert phytoestrogens into their active form. A probiotic supplement will be helpful here.

The two most potent phytoestrogens are flaxseeds and soy, and the products made from it like tofu, miso and tempeh. Some people don't get on with soy but most, in my clinical experience, do well with flaxseeds.

Practical takeaway: Try tofu, not just once, but have a go at a few different recipes. The marinated and smoked versions are very nice, and tofu in general works well scrambled (like you would an egg), in smoothies (go for silken tofu) or cubed and added to stir fries. Flaxseeds might seem easier. Top yoghurt with 1 tbsp flaxseeds, chuck in a smoothie or sprinkle on a salad or soup (try it before you judge).

Stinky veg

This is not an official term but consider smelly veg to be literally any veg that smells when you cook it: broccoli, cauliflower, cabbage, Brussels sprouts, spring greens (aka collard greens), kale, kohlrabi, onions, leeks, swede, turnip, plus several others like rocket, watercress, radish, and horseradish. These are great for women's health thanks largely to the glucosinolates they contain. They boast two sulphur-containing compounds sulforaphane and diindolylmethane (aka DIM) that help the liver recycle old oestrogens.

Practical takeaway: If you can get in a couple of servings a day, that's a very good thing. Over to you.

Eat a variety & make it colourful

In real life, so many foods can be helpful in keeping you healthy and in good shape for their vitamin and mineral, and phytonutrient content. Eating a wide variety of different foods over the course of the week - and by this I mean animal and plant foods - is the best way to get all the raw materials your body needs and to keep a healthy gut since all the different bacteria like something different for dinner. I know this is a bit dull, but there you have it. There isn't a magic pill.

One of the easiest ways to improve your health in general is to eat more plants, and this is widely agreed by all nutritional scientists. You don't have to turn vegan. All fruit and veg, plus herbs and spices, nuts and seeds, beans and lentils and so on, are plant foods. They're high in vitamins and minerals, and also the polyphenols your gut loves. The different colours are all meaningful for your health so eat the rainbow of colours through the week to ensure you get the full benefits because the plant chemicals in them work synergistically. The sum is greater than the individual components. 30 different plants a week is easier than you think. And it's not an arbitrary number. Among other things, we know that people who eat at least 30 different plants a week have a happier gut environment.

Since we're most interested in your metabolism here, I have to tell you fibre is the *big deal* in plants as it slows down the release of sugars in starchy carbs like bread, rice and pasta. This impacts how full you feel, how energised, and improves insulin sensitivity. The fibre also helps keep you regular. You know what I mean. It makes logical sense that getting waste and toxins out of your body is a good thing. Is it just me, but are there few things so satisfying as a good poo?

> **10-second recap**
> There are no foods that will - even if you eat them all together - make as big a difference to your metabolism as getting the food strategy right (discussed in previous chapters) but these foods, for one reason or another can help in a small way: green tea, coffee, ginger, chilli, turmeric, rhubarb, 'sirt foods', cinnamon, phytoestrogens like soy and flaxseeds, and all stinky veg (veg that has a strong smell when you cook it).

CHAPTER 9
HOW TO EAT

If you've been following along from the beginning, you'll know how metabolism goes all kinds of wrong in midlife and some of the things that can help you fix it. Chief among them is doing the food work. You absolutely *have to* do the food work, which is what this entire section of the book is all about. But it's not just *what* you eat that matters. How matters, too, and in this chapter, I'll be giving you another few aces to have up your sleeve. These are helpful for anyone wanting to lose weight but they really matter if you're a woman over 40. As a bonus, they are all pretty easy to do - even if you've not done them before. What are they? Eating your food in a specific order (where you can, I mean; don't be weird about it), eating more mindfully and not eating at all sometimes aka fasting). The latter, though it might sound terrifying and scream 'restricted diet' is something you are literally doing while you sleep, so breathe easy.

Food order

This is exactly what it sounds like. The order in which you eat changes how your body responds to it. Think about what you know from your time here with me.

- Some foods (anything with sugars, most refined foods and starchy carbs) will spike your blood sugars and this is not a good thing when you do it too often. These foods also lead to blood sugar drops that cause cravings and make you feel hungry.

- Some foods (fibre and protein) slow down how quickly sugars enter your bloodstream, causing fewer spikes.
- Some foods (again, fibre and protein) keep you feeling fuller for longer so naturally minimise your desire to snack.

It's great for your health to focus your diet, as already discussed, on lean proteins, veggies, fruit, healthy fats and slow-releasing wholegrains in smaller amounts. But sometimes we don't want to. Sometimes there is a buffet to be eaten or a big birthday dinner or even just date night. Or whatever. And you want what you want. This is when the food order trick can be really helpful.

Imagine you have a plate of steak, fries and veg or salad, eat the veg first, then the steak and, finally, the fries. Here's why:

The veggies (or have a generous salad if you'd rather) contain fibre and this slows down the speed at which everything else lands in your bloodstream. Most veggies contain little to impact your blood glucose and, instead, they form a kind of fibrous net in the small intestine that slows gastric emptying, which means any starchy foods eaten afterwards create less of a blood sugar spike than they otherwise would.

Next, you'll eat the steak and any fats (replace steak with chicken or fish, eggs, tofu, nuts and seeds, depending on your preference but the point is it's protein after the veggies). The protein and fat also slow down how quickly the starchy carbs or sugars enter your bloodstream. They're the next line of 'defence' against a spike after that fibrous net of veggies.

Lastly, tuck into the fries (or insert your own starchy carb preference). Since the veggies, proteins and fats are slowing down how quickly the glucose molecules hit your bloodstream (and it's the speed that dictates the size of the spike and the corresponding dip), there is less impact on your metabolism.

This is the reason it's always better to have dessert rather than a sweet snack, by the way. If you eat a bar of chocolate or a muffin on its own, it's not going to go so well for your blood sugar control. After you've eaten a full meal, the sugars hit your bloodstream more slowly. You might even have seen on Instagram people eating chocolate bars and measuring their blood glucose levels with a continuous glucose monitor, then running the experiment again but eating a serving of broccoli just before the chocolate. Different story, with far less of a spike.

When you eat veggies, meat/ protein/ fat *then* your starches, you win. You're still eating the same meal, but the impact on your metabolism is a different ball game.

Eating food in a certain order minimises the impact of 'special' meals but it won't always be possible so don't fret. I wouldn't expect you to pick the meat out of the lasagne or a risotto but if you are eating something like this, have a generous salad with it and eat it before, then eat the lasagne or risotto as the cook intended. You won't be far off the mark. Sometimes this advice might seem just too much, and that's also OK.

Go for a walk

Granny was right, a gentle walk after dinner is a good thing for your health, and part of the reason is because you are immediately putting to use some of the glucose you have just consumed. Rather than sitting down to watch Netflix after dinner, get the plates in the dishwasher then head out for a 10-minute walk. I'm not talking here about walking to burn calories or get your heart rate up. You've just had dinner and no one needs that. But the act of walking requires muscles to be used, and muscles are like glucose sponges. When you move, they use up the glucose in your bloodstream. You don't have to dash out immediately after a meal. Any time within the hour works, since your glucose will peak about an hour or so after finishing a meal.

On summer evenings, this might feel do-able but, I get it, it's not going to happen on a cold, dark, rainy winter evening. If you want to try this trick, any kind of movement works. It doesn't have to be a workout. You could choose just to go up and down the stairs for a bit. Would you do it at every meal? Of course not. Do it when you can and you want to and if it makes sense and especially after a meal that is heavier in the starches department. It makes most sense for midlife women to keep a handle on their starches for all sorts of reasons I discussed but sometimes there is pudding and this is a good way of using up that excess energy before it gets stored around your middle.

Mindful eating

The vast majority of people don't really focus on what they're eating - or maybe I should say *that* they are eating. They're throwing breakfast in their face as they dash out to work, inhaling a pasta salad before they go into a meeting or snaffling a bag of crisps in the car on the way to take the cat to the vet, and then it's their evening meal on a tray in front of the TV. Insert your own circumstances but you get the picture.

This ability to sandwich a couple of minutes of eating (sorry about the pun) between other commitments is convenient and that somehow makes it feel like your friend.

But it's not. I'm betting you do more of this mindless eating than you do fully concentrating on your meals. Everyone does. You're in a world of something entirely different that might be the grocery shopping list or working out some important life equation and then you look down at your plate and wonder where the meal went. I believe that eating in this semi-conscious way is what's lurking behind many of the health problems people experience – not to mention the number on the scale climbing north.

There are all kinds of things that just don't work when these scenarios are playing out so let's talk about that for a moment.

Your stomach doesn't have teeth and, if you're wolfing down your chow so quickly, you're probably not doing a lot of chewing. It's much more likely that these things will happen:

- Indigestion
- Bloating
- Trapped wind/ gas

Although you have spent years training yourself to eat without a second's thought, there are actually a lot of mechanics that go into eating. To summarise really quickly, digestion begins with your senses when you look at food. It gets your digestive juices flowing, then you chew it all up, your meal gets broken down in the stomach by hydrochloric acid before heading to the small intestine to be absorbed and then onwards to the large intestine and out the other end. When you skip looking and thinking about your food, and you don't chew as well as you could, food breaks down less well and you feel the discomfort at your leisure.

Perhaps the more important thing is that, if you're not present, it makes it much more likely you won't appreciate the food you've eaten - and your body might not register it much either. It's far easier to eat more than you need, and more than your body feels comfortable with.

Consider, you were born with an instinct for how much to eat, but you have become disconnected to that feeling. You've un-learnt to read your body's signals, and you're not sure you always trust yourself around food.

So let's just slow the thing down for a moment.

One of the easiest ways to avoid overeating and reduce cravings (once you've fixed your blood glucose levels) is by practising mindful eating. Now wait, before you start to think I'm going to ask you to spend 20 minutes meditating on a single raisin, let me be clear what I mean and why it's a good thing for you to try.

Yes, all mindful eating means is eating slowly and without distraction. It is also eating with intention and bringing an awareness to the process so that you can gain an understanding of when and why you eat. This in itself can be a huge catalyst for changing habits. That might sound a bit woo woo. It's not. Think of mindful eating as eating with the intention of caring for yourself and with the attention needed so that you can enjoy your food more. It really is the key to the kingdom because you begin to teach your brain to once again listen to your body and unlearn the unhelpful habits related to what, when and how you eat.

If you give yourself a teeny bit of time, mindful eating is easy. It's just something you might not have done before. It will allow you to naturally regain control around food but it is definitely not a new way to cut calories or otherwise limit what you are eating, earning or deserving or being rewarded with food, cutting out food groups, or a new way to judge yourself about what you eat or how you do it.

Mindful eating is a skill. It's not hard but you will have to push past all the stuff you did in the past. I'm going to give you an exercise to try in a moment but I don't want you to overthink it. This mindful eating lark is simply focussing your attention on the experience of eating your food and not doing anything else. At all. Fancy giving this a go? I hope so.

How to eat mindfully

Once you have the other food work sorted - or you could start here but don't try to juggle both new concepts at once - for one week, choose one meal to be a 'mindful meal' in which you will deliberately slow down. That's step one.

Note: the goal is just one meal a day and not more. It doesn't really matter when it is but you're most likely to have success with breakfast or lunch since you can often choose to eat this away from others, and the evening meal for many is more of a social occasion. It also doesn't need to be the same meal every day.

Essentially, you are zoning in on the business of eating, recognising all the textures and flavours in that meal. Your mind will wander off, and you will find yourself thinking other thoughts like 'What about the car MOT?' and 'Did I put the washing on?' This is normal. Just gently bring it back.

Here it is step by step:

1. STOP Before you eat, take a couple of seconds to tune into your environment and with your desire to eat. Be curious, not judgey.
2. RELAX Sit yourself down at the table and shake out your shoulders to relax. Everything is exactly the way it should be right now. Remember, you are learning and practising new things :)
3. REMOVE DISTRACTIONS Choose a quiet time to eat, ideally when you are alone so you can really focus. Put your phone on silent and don't have it at the table so you're not tempted by WhatsApp notifications and the like.
4. SET A TIMER Give yourself a certain amount of time to eat your meal. 20 minutes is a good start. It probably won't take you that amount of time; you're just removing the need to do anything else during this task.
5. LOOK at your meal. Notice the colours on your plate, the shape of the foods and any other physical properties. Don't judge your plate – no food is inherently good or bad. If you notice any judgement, bring your mind back to the food properties.
6. SMELL Deep breath in. Notice the aroma for a while. Really take it in.
7. TAKE THE FIRST BITE Close your eyes and take your first bite. Notice how it feels in your mouth; the texture, the taste. Where do you notice the flavour? Does it feel hot or cold? Chew until your mouthful is thoroughly soft, then swallow.
8. CONTINUE TO EAT You can open your eyes after you've had that first bite but continue to eat mindfully.

After a few bites, your mind will probably start to wander. There's nothing wrong; just notice the tendency to do this. Bring your thoughts back to your meal and the experience of eating. Your mind may drift a number of times and that's okay. The point of mindful eating - just like meditating - is not to win an Olympic medal for it.

You're not doing it for the *achievement* as such, but for the experience. This isn't about eating less, though you may in time start to notice yourself getting full so you naturally want to stop eating. This is okay. The exercise is not a cunning ploy to have you cut your calories. Simply that, when you eat mindfully you experience the meal more fully, and it will, therefore, feel more satisfying.

> ### Tricia's story
> When I asked Tricia to try mindful eating, she was sceptical that something so low-tech would make a difference but she'd been experiencing a lot of bloating and fatigue and figured she had nothing to lose by giving it a go.
>
> She chose lunch as her one mindful meal and the results of her experiment were impressive. Within a few days she told me she'd noticed a big difference in the amount of bloating. Her score before the experiment was 4 on a scale of 1 to 6, which dropped to 1 by the end of her mindful eating week. She also noted feeling more satisfied with the food she was eating and enjoying it more. She still has a mindful meal every lunch and has made it a 'rule' that she always eats at a table.

Fasting

I am a big fan of fasting because it is about *not* doing something rather than doing something and my life often feels so chaotic and full that not doing something is a blessed relief.

Essentially, fasting is not eating for a set period of time. There are lots of different types of fasts and they vary in length and intensity. For the purposes of this book, I'm going to be talking about the kind of fasting I most often use with my clients. It's effective and clients tell me it's easy to and it fits nicely into their lives. It's a type of fasting called Time Restricted Eating, and it involves squishing the food you do eat into a smaller eating 'window'. I'll explain more in a moment but let's get a couple of things straight before we plough on. The point of fasting is not 'skipping a meal'. It is not done to cut calories per se, although you might end up doing so. Done correctly, fasting can be very good for your health and is one of the most powerful things you can do for your midlife metabolism. However, I have also had clients come to work with me who have been doing all the things to lose weight in their 40s and 50s, including adopting fasts of 16+ hours and have ended up cutting calories too far, making their body go into survival mode and this is the opposite of what we want.

If you already know you don't want to do any fasting, it isn't a deal-breaker. I think it can be a valuable tool for perimenopausal, menopausal and otherwise midlife women but it isn't a biggie if you're giving this a hard no. You're very welcome to skip to the next section of the book, or maybe stay a while and hear what I have to say even if you're not yet convinced.

Let's get the housekeeping out of the way first…

Who cannot fast?

Everyone can fast to some extent. Unless there is a particular medical reason, we should all have at least equal periods of eating and not eating because - as you will soon learn - a lot of important work goes on when you are not eating. So that means 12 hours in which to eat your meals and 12 hours of not eating. That is safe for everyone.

Fasting that extends beyond this - which is what I really mean when I write 'fasting' - is not for everyone. There are some groups of people for whom fasting is not a good idea:

- You should not fast if you are pregnant or breastfeeding. Nutritional needs are significantly increased during pregnancy and breastfeeding to support the growth and development of the baby and for maternal health. You may scoff as this is a book for midlifers but a good friend, at the tender age of 48, thought she was deep in

perimenopause since her period had stopped but it turns out she was having a surprise baby. It happens.
- If you have a history of eating disorders, do not fast. Fasting can trigger eating disorder symptoms or exacerbate existing ones. For those who've struggled with anorexia, bulimia, binge eating disorder, or other related conditions, fasting may promote an unhealthy relationship with food and body image.
- If you are already underweight, again it's a no. This is anyone with a Body Mass Index (BMI) under 18.5 since fasting could lead to further weight loss, which might result in malnutrition and other health problems.
- Do you have a diagnosed medical condition? If you do, check with your doctor before you undertake any radical changes to your diet and lifestyle like fasting. I'm thinking here of people already diagnosed with diabetes or on medications for blood sugar regulation who could experience low blood sugar levels during fasting. Also ask your doctor if you have other health conditions like low blood pressure, heart disease, kidney disease, or liver disease. Some mental health conditions, such as bipolar disorder and depression, might worsen with fasting due to changes in the body's production of hormones and neurotransmitters. This is obviously not an exhaustive list. If in doubt, check with the doc.
- Are you stressed? I'll be talking more about this in the next part of the book because it's BIG for perimenopausal women but if you know you are stressed already, don't extend a fast much beyond 12 hours. Like exercise, fasting is considered a positive stressor, which means that, though it is good for your health, it does exert a little more stress on your body and this will not be helpful. Skip this step and focus on the food and the lifestyle aspects. When you're feeling strong, fasting will always be here for you.

Different types of fasting

We're going to be talking about time restricted eating (TRE) but just to fill you in, there are many different fasting regimes. I think you'll probably see why TRE is the easiest for most women to accommodate.

Intermittent fasting is often used interchangeably with TRE, although strictly it's a little different although they both involve periods of eating and fasting. What is different is the timing and duration of fasting periods.

Some common ways of doing intermittent fasting are:
- **5:2 Method:** involves eating normally for five days of the week and restricting calories to about 800 for the remaining two days. The late, great Dr Michael Mosely made this approach popular.
- **Alternate-Day Fasting:** involves eating normally one day and either completely fasting or severely restricting calories the next day.
- **Eat-Stop-Eat:** involves a 24-hour fast once or twice a week.

Then there is TRE. This method restricts your daily eating window to a certain number of hours. When people talk about a 14-hour fast they mean 14 hours of not eating, and a 'window' of 10 hours during which you can eat. This is the timeframe I use most frequently with clients and, maybe because of its rhythmic nature, people seem to find it both easy and enjoyable, and of course they reap the health benefits.

You might also hear people talk about a 20-hour fast. I think that is not a great idea as a regular thing for women. Or even OMAD, which stands for 'one meal a day'.

There are folk who make it their business to only eat one giant meal every day. I do not advocate it for women for various reasons and here are some important things to know:
- Longer fasts (beyond about 14 hours) can be too much and too hard on the body. You will learn more about stress in the next section. Suffice to say for now, too much stress will sabotage any efforts of weight loss and/ or metabolism fixing. It will directly work against you.
- Often, I will find very strong, capable, and high-achieving women who are used to having to push boundaries in so many aspects of their life will try to go for the longer fasts but it ends up working against them. There are plenty of metabolic benefits from a 14- hour fast. You don't need to routinely go beyond this.

- Occasionally, a longer fast can be helpful but it must be used strategically. Women are cyclical creatures and at some stages in your cycle (if you are still cycling) your body will not enjoy the fasting process so much. If you have ever tried fasting but crashed and burned, you may well have tried it at the wrong time in your cycle (if you are still cycling). You have to work with your body. You cannot bend your metabolism to your will.

Fasting of one kind or another is an important part of fixing your midlife metabolism - but remember, it's not the be all and end all and to what extent midlife women should fast is a complicated business - and this means it really deserves its own chapter, so see you on the next page…

10-second recap

How you eat matters as well as what you eat, and there are a variety of different tools you can employ to help enhance your midlife metabolism. Food order (veggies, then protein and, lastly, starchy carbs) can help you avoid a blood glucose spike. A post-meal walk can also help here. Mindful eating reduces overeating. Fasting can increase sensitivity to the fat storage hormone insulin, so you'll naturally make less of it but take care it's not too much for your midlife body.

CHAPTER 10
MAKE FASTING WORK FOR YOU

Fasting can be a game changer but it is not the golden ticket. You must tread carefully in menopause to ensure you get the benefits, and this is what this chapter is all about.

Let's make one thing clear, fasting is not code for 'starving'. Fasting is a choice – voluntarily choosing not to eat for health and sometimes spiritual reasons. It's an entirely natural process. Fasting is nothing new - although it's been somewhat forgotten until the last decade - yet it's probably the oldest and most powerful dietary intervention with huge therapeutic potential. Human beings have fasted for millennia without detrimental consequences to health so don't believe any scare stories. There were times when food was plentiful and there were times when food was scarce. The human body evolved to adapt to these cycles of feast and fast. There is a certain irony that many women dedicate their lives to finding the 'best' diet for them and, by the time they hit menopause, it turns out that the best diet might involve periods of not eating at all.

There is a lot of science around fasting but I want you to keep in mind these things:

1. What you eat when you are eating matters - fasting cannot undo the harm caused by a poor diet.
2. Fasting should not be used as a highway to undereating. This will wreck your metabolism.
3. Longer is not better, and long fasts *will* work against you if you're stressed or not sleeping enough.

4. Breaking your fast earlier in the day is probably better in midlife than going straight to lunch.
5. You should always listen to your body. You are the expert in being you. If you've tried fasting and felt weak or depleted, something is not right and you should stop.

This is how fasting heals a broken metabolism

These are some of the important things you learnt earlier that explain the beauty of fasting for healing your metabolism.

- Many people have spent too long eating sugars and starchy carbs, and the body can only take so much of the strain without starting to malfunction. This shows up as impaired glucose function (too much glucose in the blood) and insulin resistance, which in turn creates the situation in which the body makes too much insulin in response to the foods you eat, keeping you overweight, inflamed, and starving. Yes, this is an oversimplification, but a decent one.
- When you don't eat, the body does not have to make insulin. It gets a break.
- Since the body needs energy whether you are sleeping or at a yoga class, it must use its own resources - all your stored fat - as fuel. There is nearly always plenty of it. First, it runs down the sugars in your bloodstream, then it goes looking for energy stored in the liver and muscles (this is called glycogen), after that is used up, it will tap into your fat stores. As a side note, your body finds it easy to run down the energy stored in your muscles. It can get to that from exercise. But the fat that gets stored around the liver and in your fat cells? That's much trickier to get at without fasting, and that's one of the reasons fasting is so great.
- When you fast, your body releases excess glucose and excess insulin. Remember, insulin resistance happens when your cells are flooded with insulin, so releasing it is a good thing. The more you put your body into a fasted state, the more your body is forced to find those hidden stores of energy.

Benefits of fasting

No question, fasting is very good for your metabolic health, but there are many other positive benefits reported by those who fast regularly. These include:

- Cellular repair (autophagy)
- More energy
- Increased mental clarity and reduced brain fog
- Lower insulin and blood sugar levels
- Lowered cholesterol
- Reduction in inflammation
- Better digestion
- Faster recovery after exercise
- Better immunity
- Lower risk of cancer
- Slower ageing
- Improved brain function and lower risk of dementia

Longer fasts

Since this isn't a book on fasting, and longer fasts are best done with a measure of supervision, I'm just going to mention in passing that there can sometimes be merit in longer fasts but whether it's a good idea for midlife women like you is debatable. There may be subclinical medical situations - like impaired thyroid function - or it might be too much stress for your body to handle. But it would be remiss of me not to tell you that sometimes there is a reason to fast for a longer period.

The main reasons for a longer fast are to switch on a process called autophagy and for a speedier reset for insulin resistance. But, I'll say this again, the stress hormone cortisol is a big deal in menopause and midlife so don't be tempted to do a long fast if you suspect stress may be playing anything other than a bit part in your life. It will really work against you and negate any metabolic gain fasting may give you. One further note, this kind of longer fasting is an occasional fast, not a thing to do every day - just for the few who will ignore the above advice anyway.

The risks of fasting in midlife

Fasting is a stressor, but often a positive one. Generally speaking, the longer the fast, the more the stress - and this is the issue in the menopause years. When you get to midlife, your baseline stress hormones are higher, and if you exercise hard (even when you're doing the 'right' exercise for this life stage), that too is a stressor. If you exercise in a fasted state, you're adding stress on top of stress. And if long fasts mean you're dropping your calories too low, this is also bad news because women are more sensitive to energy restriction than men, and this can disrupt your hormones.

There are conflicting theories on fasting in perimenopause and the science is changing all the time. Over time, my stance, too, has changed but here's my take right now on fasting.

My 'rules' on fasting

- Some fasting is good and I think everyone should have 12 hours fasting so there's a balance between being fed and giving your body a rest. If you can do 14 hours, perfect.
- If you've been used to pushing your breakfast later in the day to get your fasting hours in, you might want to look at your schedule again. An earlier breakfast is likely to be better for you right now coupled with an earlier evening meal. The reason lies in your stress hormones.
- Since stress hormones are highest in the morning (the stress hormone cortisol in women peaks half an hour after you wake up), this puts you in a stressed state from the off (this is sometimes called a fight or flight or a 'sympathetic' state). A long fast can exacerbate that stress, so eating an hour after waking up will lift your blood sugar levels a little, signalling to the body that there's some food on board and you're good to start your day, which allows cortisol to drop.
- Exercising is good but the latest science suggests midlife women might be better not exercising in a fasted state (and worse still fasted after coffee) as this adds further stress and can disrupt production of oestrogen and progesterone and downregulate thyroid function. If

you like to workout first thing, jiggle your schedule so you can have a small breakfast (even if it's a protein shake) 30 minutes to an hour before working out.

I'll leave you to work out the logistics but know this: 12 to 14 hours is a great start. Don't let this small piece stress you out. If you cannot fathom how to get this to work, let it go. Eat three meals a day and don't snack in between. And do all the other stuff but discount this one small piece of the puzzle.

How to get started with fasting

If you know your diet has not been great recently, if you're a big snacker or you eat late at night, start with a 12-hour fast to bring things back into line very gently. Do this every day for a week, eating three meals a day and no snacks in between. This isn't really 'fasting'. It's what every human should be doing to give their body some time off.

Next, I want you to go with a 14-hour fast (you eat in a ten-hour window so the ratio of fasting to eating looks like 14:10), again eating three meals but no snacks. It might not be that different from what you're currently doing. In practice, that might mean having dinner at 6pm and then eating your breakfast at 8am the next morning, after waking up around 7am.

During your eating window, eat real food using the strategies set out earlier in the book, and do the lifestyle work (which we'll talk about in the next section) so that you are giving yourself the best chance of your body working optimally.

What you can eat & drink when fasting

You cannot consume anything that is 'food' when you fast. It's a given the cheeseburger is out but so too is 'food' you drink - like your morning latte (milk is food even though it's liquid, and the natural sugars will break your fast). Ideally, you would drink only water, black tea and black coffee. You'll consume no calories at all in the fasting period and ideally also no zero calorie cheats like diet fizzy drinks/ soda.

The former is what the fasting community calls 'clean' fasting. The latter, 'dirty' fasting, and it includes artificially sweetened drinks, bone broth, a little high fat cream in your coffee, or 'bulletproof' coffee (the kind of coffee with butter and/ or MCT oil – yes, I thought that sounded gross when I first heard it too). Some people believe this makes fasting more manageable, but others argue it could interrupt the fasting state. It's worth mentioning that there's ongoing debate and research about whether the small amounts of calories in a dirty fast significantly impact the benefits of fasting. Different people might also have different responses to clean versus dirty fasting. We'll let them thrash that one out. My recommendation? Stick to water and herbal tea and drown out the noise.

You must stay well hydrated during your fast. At least 2 litres of water minimum. There are a multitude of benefits to drinking more water but, for now, know that drinking more water will help squish your hunger pangs.

When you have been fasting, your insulin levels are very low and the body has been using your stored fat as energy. To continue to burn fat after you close your fasting window by beginning to eat, you should eat a lowish carb diet (but not no carb), just like the one I describe, so that there is less sugar in the blood for the body to use and store. It will, therefore, find it far easier to dip into your fat stores.

Right now, especially if your diet hasn't been anything like the kind of thing I've been talking about in this book, and you've been riding that blood sugar rollercoaster, the thought of not eating may sound terrifying. When you get your body back into balance by eating the kinds of foods your metabolism loves, it will feel easier.

Keep in mind, the reason fasting is so good has nothing to do with calories but with your metabolic health. When you optimise your eating window, you improve your insulin sensitivity. When you have good insulin sensitivity, your body becomes metabolically flexible - able to effectively use both carbs and fat for fuel - and that is the gold.

Rachel's story

Rachel started working with me because her menopausal symptoms – such as brain fog - were getting out of hand and she was frustrated she wasn't losing weight. She was deeply invested in fasting but, although the lengthy fasts sounded like the golden ticket, they were actually working against her. One of the things we worked on was gently increasing the number of calories she was eating as long fasts had shrunk her eating window so far that she was under-eating and her body had gone into energy-conservation mode. We brought breakfast forward, introducing a protein smoothie first thing that made it easy to get her metabolism up and running after an overnight fast so she could also do her morning exercise.

'At first, the thought of doing this was terrifying,' she told me. 'I was convinced that long fasts and cutting calories were going to save me and it was just a matter of time. I'd assumed that, when things weren't working the way I wanted, it was my fault, that I must be doing something wrong or I just needed to keep going.'

By the end of her 12-week programme, things had changed. Her brain fog and anxiety had diminished, and the number on the scales was well and truly headed in the right direction.

10-second recap

Everyone should have a 12-hour gap between the last meal of the evening and the first meal of the next day, and that includes not consuming drinks that contain milk. The reason is that the body needs time to rest and repair. There are many benefits to fasting and most of them are achieved with a 14-hour fast. In midlife, long fasts can be problematic as they place additional stress on your body so eat an hour or two after waking up, have a small breakfast before you work out, and finish eating earlier in the day. Above all, don't stress if this approach feels genuinely unworkable in your life.

PART THREE

CHAPTER 11
SLEEP, THE REAL GAME CHANGER

The 'lifestyle work' is a MUST in midlife. Yes, the food is critical but getting more zen is too. Sometimes, I even work on my clients' lifestyle first because, if you're stressed, knackered and miserable, the cake and crisps will always win.

Fixing your sleep is where I'd start.

If you're convinced you are 'doing everything right' and yet you're still not getting the results you want or that other people you know have had, poor sleep might well be the reason. Restorative sleep is an essential part of life yet we seem to think it's OK to scrape by with as little of the stuff as possible, and we do this for years and years.

Hardly anyone I know sleeps enough. We are in an epidemic of busyness and sleep deprivation and it's not only making your menopause worse, it's wrecking your metabolism and every conceivable area of your health.

I know *you* know on a conceptual level at least that you should get more sleep. There will be times when you've had a great sleep and felt you could conquer the world and other times when you've not slept well and you've felt grouchy and hungry all day. Yet somehow sleep never gets to be the priority it deserves.

Knowing you should get more sleep is the same as knowing you should drink more water. Both are free and you could do more of either - in theory at least - at any time. But there's no urgency and it feels an oversimplification of health because we've become accustomed to having to pay for the privilege of transforming the way we feel.

Or maybe you would love it if only you *could* only sleep more. According to the Sleep Foundation, 40% of women over 40 struggle with sleep, compared to 12% of younger women; a dramatic increase.

So, this chapter is all about sleep and why you need it, and I'm hoping you'll soon be able to look at sleep with a fresh pair of eyes and create an action plan to get more of this elixir into your life so that you can feel fabulous. Sounds cheesy, but this is what is at stake.

The women I've met in clinic or who have otherwise spoken to me about their sleep - like at a dinner party or in the queue at the supermarket (it happens) - will usually fall into one of these categories:

1. The hot flushes and night sweats make sleeping through the night impossible. These are often accompanied by random wakings. The symptoms are sometimes helped by HRT but, if you're already on HRT and haven't had the breakthrough you were hoping for, the following scenario might also apply.
2. They fall asleep easily but wake in the middle of the night - usually about 3am - and can't easily get back to sleep. While occasionally they do drop back off, sometimes sleep eludes them for hours on end. This is usually linked to poor blood glucose control.
3. They struggle to fall asleep. As soon as their head hits the pillow, it fills with thoughts of things they should do or else they start raking over the ashes of the day. They will sleep at some stage but it could take an hour or more. This is linked to stress hormone imbalance.
4. They just don't have enough time to get eight hours of sleep on a regular basis. This is a diary issue.

Sleep: why you need it and how much you need

Far from your body just powering off overnight, there is a lot going on when you sleep, and scientific knowledge is deepening all the time. Sleep is when your body gets to rest and repair and that process takes between seven and nine hours a night, which is where that magic number of 'eight hours' comes in. This is what science tells us you need each night, regardless of what you may have trained yourself to get by on. The quality of your sleep is also important. It is not enough to be geographically in your bed.

A lot of what scientists know about the benefits of sleep comes from research into what happens when you don't get enough of it. You probably know first-hand about the poor concentration, lack of creativity and loss of productivity that comes from not getting enough shut-eye. Peak performance is not possible if you've not slept well. Aside from many other actions, did you know that sleep removes toxins in your brain that build up while you're awake, so small wonder getting your fill makes you feel more alive and your head less cluttered.

The extra 'bonus' you get with poor sleep is that all your relationships suffer. That includes the relationship you have with yourself, which is vital for women as they age. You're also just not that great to be around either, and other people pick up on that vibe you're giving off. If you think I'm making this up, consider that one study found people lacking in the sleep department were less attractive and looked less healthy than more rested folk, which made others want to give them a wide berth.

Many people find it hard to take seriously the idea of preventative medicine, which is acting now in order to avoid ill health at some unknown point in the future, and I really do get it. It's human nature not to feel motivated to take action where there's not enough of a problem in the here-and-now.

But what I'm going to tell you next might really hit home.

My clients are women in their 40s and beyond, and one of the things that bothers them most about their health is weight gain, and specifically the kind that doesn't seem to shift no matter what they try. That comes down to hormones and metabolism. If you are ever looking for a magic pill for weight loss (among a great many other things), sleep is probably it.

However you feel about sleep and how much you're getting, I want you to think of sleep as a game. It's a game of hormones and getting the right ones in the right amounts at the right time. When something is off, your sleep quality is negatively affected. But - to a greater extent than you realise - how well you sleep is under your control.

Hormones are the chemical messengers in your body. Lack of sleep messes up those messages, but there are lots of ways to hack your hormones with some simple lifestyle tricks so your body gets what it needs.

The 'right' amount of sleep is very individual. Only you will know what's right for you. And by that I don't mean how much you can get or what you are currently surviving on. With a little trial, error and general practice, you can figure out the magic number for you that genuinely has you feeling and looking your best. Measuring your general mood is probably a good indicator.

Problem: flushes and general menopause unrest

In perimenopause, the 'sleep piece' will almost certainly have reared its ugly head because how well you'll sleep at certain ages is partly dictated by your lady hormones. As you get older, sleep can get a bit scrappy for this reason alone. The hot flushes and night sweats caused by falling levels of oestrogen are enough to keep anyone from restful slumber. What happens is that changes in your brain combined with that sudden feeling of hotness trigger sleep disturbances.

If you're in that post-menopause territory, it's also more likely (compared with premenopausal) you'll suffer from something called sleep apnoea, a sleep disorder that results in frequent nighttime wakings, as a result of which you're totally exhausted. It's another of your body's survival instincts that don't work so well in our modern lives.

Here's the short version of what you need to know about sleep apnoea. Younger women are protected – thanks to higher levels of lady hormones – because oestrogen and progesterone help maintain muscle tone in your airway as you sleep. If your airway collapses during the night, this obstruction causes more frequent pauses in breathing or shallow breathing. The survival reflex wakes you up in enough time for you to resume breathing.

Another thing you'll want to know is that oestrogen allows your body to better use the 'happy hormone' serotonin, which is the precursor to the 'sleep hormone' melatonin. During menopause, when oestrogen levels fall steadily, the lack of progesterone (which practically falls off a cliff) is problematic because progesterone helps you fall asleep faster and experience fewer disruptions to your sleep.

Solution: it doesn't matter if you are on HRT or not, diet and lifestyle is the big game changer for your sleep.

Sleep stages

I'm not going to go on too long about sleep stages but I think it will help you understand why you might be waking up in the middle of the night. The sleep cycle is made up of several different stages, and you'll cycle through all of them a number of times each night. The exact pattern will change from person to person and even from day to day. If you have a smart watch with an app that measures your sleep cycles or a smart ring, you probably know this already. Some days you'll spend longer in those deep and restorative sleep cycles than others. A complete sleep cycle takes about 90 minutes, and you'll typically go through four to five cycles each night. The normal pattern is N1, N2, N3, N2, REM.

Stage N1 (non-REM) is the lightest sleep. Your body starts to relax and brain, heart rate and breathing activity begin to slow. You might get the occasional twitch as your muscles prepare for proper sleep. You can be easily woken. Think "catnap". If you're not disturbed, you'll move into the next sleep stage.

Stage N2 (non-REM) is also fairly light. Your muscles relax further, your breathing slows as does your heart rate. Body temperature also lowers. Think "power nap". It's the sleep stage you'll probably spend most time in.

Stage N3 (non-REM) is your deepest sleep and the most restorative. It's the most difficult to wake from and, for some people, even loud noises do not rouse them. It's here that the body repairs, builds bone and muscle, and the immune system is strengthened. It is also the stage in which sleepwalking, night terrors, and bedwetting happens. If you're woken in this phase, you'll likely feel dazed and confused for a few minutes while you adjust.

Stage four is called REM sleep. REM stands for Rapid Eye Movement and this sleep stage is not usually considered a restful state with reason. The brain is very active.

Your eyes do literally dart about and your muscles are temporarily paralysed. It's the sleep phase in which you are most likely to dream, and it's important for learning, creativity, memory, and mood. This is the phase of sleep that gets trashed by booze. While drinking alcohol makes you fall asleep faster, it messes with your sleep cycle and REM sleep in particular.

According to the Sleep Foundation, you can expect a 39.2% decrease in the quality of your sleep if you have more than one drink.

Problem: waking in the middle of the night

If you have problems with your blood glucose (and many midlife women do without realising it), it's common for sugar levels to dip below a comfortable baseline during the night. This will wake you up and maybe you won't get to go back to sleep afterwards.

That's because your body has elaborate inbuilt mechanisms to keep you alive. One of these is to send in stress hormones to help increase glucose levels when your blood sugars dip too low. You don't have to be a scientist to understand that having a bunch of stress hormones in the middle of the night is a bad idea, especially if you are in a light sleep phase. You'll be cycling through light, lightish, deep and REM sleep throughout the night and, if those stress hormones come in during a light sleep, good luck with getting back off again. You'll be properly awake like it's morning. If they hit during a deep sleep, you'll be roused - maybe you'll get up for a wee - but chances are, you'll fall back to sleep again pretty quickly.

Solution: diet. I frequently find that, once my clients have got their blood sugar levels back under control with diet, this kind of nighttime waking stops. If you often find yourself waking in the middle of the night, do the diet work ASAP.

Problem: can't seem to get to sleep?

We'll delve deeper into the ticking time bomb that is stress in the next chapter but one of the main things to know is that, when your oestrogen levels drop as you move towards menopause, levels of your stress hormones are inclined to rise. Your body is designed to deal with a lot behind the scenes without creating issues but it can only tolerate so much without noticeable symptoms of one sort or another. Struggling to get to sleep - the main restorative process - is designed to make you take notice when stress levels get out of hand.

Stress doesn't have to be 'big' stuff like divorce, bereavement, or a house move. It could equally be the relentlessness of daily life – like work issues, family or relationship worries, or even traffic jams. Just thinking about something that's worrying you, or reliving a traumatic event causes stress hormones to course through your body.

Regardless of the source, stress triggers the hypothalamic-pituitary-adrenal (HPA) axis in the central nervous system and puts you in fight or flight mode; essentially, a sense of high alert. When this stress has been going on for a while, that means prolonged stimulation of this HPA axis - a situation our primitive bodies were not set up for - and, potentially, higher levels of stress hormones at night. If you've ever felt tired but wired (exhausted physically but your mind is whirring), this is it. And until you can dial down those stress hormones, you'll have little chance of nodding off.

Solution: de-stress action plan. This is coming up in a couple of chapters.

Stress & sleep hormones

The stress hormone cortisol is not a bad thing. You need cortisol, but it's important to have the right hormones in the right amounts at the right time. The stress hormone cortisol and the sleep hormone melatonin have an inverse relationship. Where one is high, the other should be low. In the morning, when you first wake up, cortisol levels should be at their peak, helping you spring out of bed. Cortisol levels should then drop throughout the day so they are nice and low, ready for bedtime. Then they begin to climb in the very early morning so they're at their peak for wakey time.

Melatonin, on the other hand, is low in the morning, stable throughout much of the day and begins to climb in the evening so it is nice and high come bedtime, peaking in the middle of the night, then tapering away such that it is low again by morning.

There is a diurnal pattern, which means a predictable, repeatable pattern that should happen reliably every day. People who have been under a lot of stress will be making more stress hormones and they can get peaks at unhelpful times.

An adrenal stress test (the best is the DUTCH test, which tests urine) gives you an idea of the pattern your cortisol levels have been following, which allows practitioners like me to get insights into why your sleep might be problematic. In people with sleep and/or energy problems, we typically see an unusual cortisol pattern. In people who are struggling to get out of bed in the morning, often morning cortisol levels are very low - you literally have no bounce. In those who feel tired but wired, we typically see elevated evening/nighttime cortisol levels.

So, the long and short of it is that, if you struggle to get off to sleep, in the absence of other obvious reasons, it might well be a cortisol issue.

Get back into balance

One thing you can start doing right now is to work better with your body's natural rhythm. That diurnal pattern? It's one of a series of clocks inside your body, in fact the most important one - the circadian rhythm, which is governed by the light and dark. You can optimise your circadian rhythm by prioritising sleep (practical ideas for how to do this coming up in the next chapter), minimising stress (that's the chapter after that), and light therapy, which basically means using nature's light/ dark cycle to benefit your chemistry. More on that in a moment.

Screens & sleep

Here comes the 'bad news' part you've been dreading. You probably read all the way through this chapter and thought, thank God she's not mentioned the late-night scrolling thing, but suddenly, here we are. Screens kill your sleep. It doesn't matter whether we're talking about smartphones, tablets, laptops, Kindles, TVs or whatnot. This might be the worst news, and I'm sorry, but the research is very clear on this.

It might seem like watching TV before bed or scrolling through your social media gets you all relaxed and in the best place for sleep but it's a trap. The blue light emitted triggers the body to produce more daytime hormones (like cortisol) and crush the release of the sleep hormone melatonin – the exact opposite of what you want.

And it's not just the light; said for the folk who have their phone set to 'night shift mode'. Screens feel like fun, and it's so hard not to end up scrolling each night. This is why: it's the tale of another hormone, and this one is called dopamine. We think of dopamine as the hormone that sends addicts into a spin over sex, drugs or shopping. Yes, dopamine is about pleasure and it is also about seeking and what's coming next. Anyone who has gone onto Instabookface, YouTube or TikTok will understand that these places are perfect for just that. One minute, you are looking at funny cat videos but the next, you've been sucked into a photo story someplace else about that actress who used to be in Eastenders and how ropey she's looking now, and suddenly the clock has moved on an hour or so. Not judging, we've all been there.

There's another problem with that hormone dopamine. Like cortisol, it's an awake hormone, which is fine during the day, but it is not OK at night for obvious reasons. In fact, it might be a good idea to banish tech from the bedroom altogether. Studies from the Loughborough University Sleep Research Centre show talking on the phone at night has a negative impact on sleep thanks to the delta rays messing with the deep sleep part of your natural sleep cycle. These waves are disrupted for more than an hour after you end the call.

There's also a lot of noise around melatonin secretion and electromagnetic fields (read 'phones'). Bottom line, consistent exposure – let's say you're keeping your phone by your bed at night as so many of us do – can throw melatonin production off.

If relying on screens at night for your entertainment has likely become ingrained in 'what you do', now would be a good time to get curious about what else you could do instead of the screens. It doesn't matter what. It might be reading a book (not on a screen), talking to your other half, taking a relaxing bath, stroking cats, some kind of gratitude or mindfulness practice, I don't know, but it must be enjoyable. Just roll that around in your head for a while.

10-second recap

Sleep is no longer something you can consider a luxury that you do if you have time. In midlife, there are a few key reasons you might be struggling to sleep. All will be helped with food and lifestyle. If you wake up in the early hours of the morning, it's likely to be a blood glucose problem, which is more easily fixed than you think.

Struggling to get to sleep is usually linked to stress or the presence of too many daytime hormones. Throwing everything you know at your sleep will improve the situation.

CHAPTER 12
HOW TO SLEEP BETTER

Annoyingly, so much of this fixing your health malarkey is a bit time consuming, and, by way of apology, I will dedicate this chapter to pulling together some of the things you might try to help with sleep and the entire fourth part of the book is dedicated to untangling what is essentially a lot of info and helping you put it into some kind of meaningful plan.

When there feels like a lot to do and a great many new things to try, working out how to get them into your already-busy life is a bit mind-blowing - and not in a good way. I believe it makes sense to create a new framework for yourself; the basic architecture of your day. This means looking at creating helpful morning and evening rituals that get you off to a good start and help you wind down properly.

Trying to work better with your circadian rhythm is a good place to start because it gets you aligned with how nature wants your life to go.

Work with your body's internal clock

The circadian rhythm is your body's internal clock, not the 'I want a baby kind' biological clock but the cycle that regulates important functions, from your sleep and the secretion and sensitivity of other hormones like insulin, to your blood pressure. Research shows bad things happen when this pattern gets disrupted, including changes to important metabolic hormones like the fat storage hormone insulin (dialled up 22%), a decrease in the satiety hormone leptin (down 17%), a flipped cortisol/ melatonin rhythm, and reduced sleep efficiency (down 20%).

So now let's have a bash at what you can do about it.

Get outdoors in the morning

Ever since the invention of the lightbulb, we've been working towards creating a 24-hour society and this messes with nature's light-dark cycle.

Your body's sleep-wake cycle is influenced by sunlight. When you expose yourself to sunlight in the morning, your body produces less melatonin during the day, which can help regulate your sleep at night. Light sensors in the retina of your eyes are the gateway. You can hack your brain chemistry by influencing the kind of light that gets in. So, sunlight in the morning, and avoiding bright lights as much as is practical in the nighttime.

Your health will really thank you for making it a habit to get outside and soak up some morning sun. I say 'sun' when we're, of course, at the mercy of the weather so let's just call it daylight. This activates cortisol in a good way, gives you energy, and sets you up for the day. Actual daylight is significantly more potent than artificial light. You cannot just put the lights on at home or look out of a window.

This is where dog walkers unwittingly have the edge. They absolutely must go out whatever the weather and the benefit is getting that early morning daylight. If you don't have a dog, your outdoor walk might involve walking to work, and, if you have a car park situation and 10 metres to your office building, consider whether you could get in that bit earlier and have a mini stroll someplace near work. You're the expert in you and know what's practical. It doesn't even have to be a walk. It could be morning boot camp, or simply sitting outside with your morning coffee. Just 10-15 minutes of exposure to sunlight can make a big difference. Another good reason to be outdoors is that sleep is also influenced by vitamin D, a hormone that is made as a result of the skin absorbing UV light.

Amy's story

Last year Amy experimented with adding a morning walk to her life and she loved it. Although she is not a 'morning person', she felt she was winning the day before she'd really begun. She started her habit in winter, pulling on a DryRobe and her walking boots so she was completely impervious to the weather around her. She loves to listen to audiobooks and every walk felt like a treat rather than a chore. She walked anything from 15 to 45 minutes, depending on when her first meeting was. There was a big impact at both ends of the day on her health. She felt more awake before work and could feel her body naturally winding down by early evening.

Dial down light in the evening

Thanks to electricity, we can choose to have lights blazing at all hours, which is not helpful for increasing melatonin. Instead, you want to encourage your body to make more of the night-time hormones, which means reducing the amount of bright light you are exposed to when the sun goes down. If you have dimmer switches on your ceiling pendants, use them to dim the main lights in the evenings. You might also consider getting someone to fit dimmers for you. It's not a big job. Or use side lights instead. These subtle lighting changes can make a difference and give your body the signal that things are getting darker so you are primed for sleep.

Get some blue light-blocking glasses

Messing with the light-dark cycle is another reason screens are not your friend. In an ideal world, you wouldn't be on your phone or tablet, or watching TV 90 minutes before bed, in part to do with the light-dark cycle and in part due to the daytime hormone trigger I talked about in the last chapter. But in practice? Do your best.

Switch screens on your phone or tablet into night shift mode when the sun goes down and consider getting some blue light-blocking glasses once you've tried all the other diet and lifestyle sleep hacks.

You might have heard of these blue light blocking glasses and wondered whether they are for you. There are different types, including the kind you can get in the opticians, which are designed to relieve eye strain and headaches. And there are the other kind, the weird ones with the orange lenses you might have seen some folk wearing, which are designed to block the kind of 'junk' blue light we get from LEDs and other artificial lights. Since light blocks the sleep hormone melatonin, they might be a good thing

- especially if you're a night owl. Will you look odd? Possibly. Will it be worth it? I think so.

Sleep in a dark room

People say 'sleep in a blacked-out room' for a reason. It works. If you can do that, great. The best night's sleep I've ever had are without doubt those when I had lovely, thick blackout curtains. If your room isn't dark and you're not sure you want to fork out on some serious blackout curtains, try a silk sleep mask. It's the next best option. Silk masks are kind to ageing skin and are very comfortable to wear. Melatonin likes the dark, and in summer, if you do wake in the early hours, you're more likely to nod back off if your sleep environment is dark compared to the full daylight summer months bring even at 5am. Get a generously-sized one that covers enough of your face to block any light getting in.

Food that helps with sleep

For good sleep, you'll want to keep your blood sugar levels steady through the day. The key to that is basing your diet on lean protein (from meat or veggie sources) and plenty of vegetables, with moderate amounts of starchy foods like bread, rice, pasta, noodles, couscous and potatoes. This prevents blood sugars spiking, then dropping too low overnight and waking you up. Remember, it's a game of hormones, and the hormone in play here is insulin. I don't need to tell you that, at a time when you might also be struggling with hot flushes and night sweats, this added risk is really not what you need.

There are many different nutrients, including amino acids, vitamins, and minerals, that are important for supporting sleep. You might have read about eating turkey before bed in a bid to get more of the amino acid tryptophan in the body, which gets turned into the 'sleep hormone' melatonin. If only it were that simple. Yes, there are some foods that are good natural sources of tryptophan, such as eggs, cheese, nuts, salmon, tofu, pineapple and that famous turkey. But it's not like popping a pill. And who actually fancies a slice of turkey at bedtime?

If you eat a balanced diet made up (most of the time) of real, unprocessed food, you'll probably be getting most of the important raw materials your body needs for good health and sleep. In case you're wondering, the following are helpful: the amino acid tryptophan, magnesium, and omega 3 fatty acids. To avoid having to overthink all the rest, eat a pretty broad diet with lean proteins, and lots of veggies and some fruit.

Coffee, tea and sleep

Caffeine is a powerful stimulant for the nervous system. Drink it and it wakes you up. You've used this to your advantage, I'm sure, on many occasions. I like coffee and I don't want to be judgemental, but you need to be the boss of caffeine if you want to win at sleeping.

When you drink caffeine, your body produces the stress (and anti-sleep) hormones adrenaline and cortisol. It also blocks adenosine receptors in the brain. This is important because the body constantly monitors for adenosine and when levels reach a certain amount, it encourages the body to get sleepy.

It's not that you can't have caffeine at all, but you must create yourself a caffeine curfew you don't stray from and learn to read your own body so that you can enjoy your morning cuppa and get a good night's sleep.

The trouble with caffeine is that it has a long half-life. That's the scientific way of describing the length of time it takes for half of a particular substance to leave your body. The half-life of caffeine is between five and eight hours, so you want to give yourself enough time to get all of it out of your system by the time you hit the pillow.

Obviously, I don't make the rules, but this applies to everyone. Even if you feel a cup of coffee after dinner at night is not stopping you getting to sleep, it *is* interfering with the quality of your sleep on some level.

One study uncovered that, when you drink caffeine six hours before bed, it could knock an hour off your sleep time (and this is actual sleep rather than the length of time you are physically in bed or in bed with your eyes shut).

The solution? Set a caffeine curfew. If you go to bed at 10pm, you'll want to have no coffee past 2pm to ensure your body on its way to being caffeine-free in time. Some people are much more sensitive to caffeine than others – it's in their genetic make-up. If you find you're the kind of person who is overstimulated by coffee, know your own body. Maybe you want to cut caffeinated drinks completely, or only take your caffeine earlier in the morning.

Alcohol & sleep

Booze is the other thing worth keeping an eye on. I hear from many of the women I work with that a few glasses of wine not only relaxes them, but that alcohol also helps them fall asleep quicker. Kind of true, and we have all been there. There have been many nights in the dark, stressful days of bereavement or divorce when a bottle of white wine felt like it was helping. And it does feel like you fall asleep quicker (the science backs this up) but your REM sleep is disrupted and, while REM is not the most restful part of your sleep, it's still critical for your wellbeing.

What also happens when you drink is, initially, alcohol sedates but after about five hours, as the sedative effects wear off, you get the opposite effect and your sleep is disrupted for the remainder of the night. Drinking alcohol also makes it more likely you'll wake in the night because you need a wee and it worsens sleep apnoea (hello, snoring). Small wonder you don't feel rested when you wake after a big night out even after a lie in.

Exercise & sleep

From a lifestyle perspective, getting outdoors is fantastic if you want to sleep well. Being outdoors in the sunshine (or even using light therapy in winter months) is known to lift levels of the 'happy hormone' serotonin, which is the warm-up act to melatonin.

It's a double whammy if you can exercise outdoors. Exercise is generally regarded as one of the best things you can do for every single aspect of your health, from balancing hormones, to keeping in shape and ensuring you stay mobile for longer.

When it comes to sleep, you'll want to make sure you're exercising (either indoors or outdoors) at the right time. Night-time exercise is not great. Exercise is a 'positive stressor' on the body, which means it's a good thing, but it also places the body under stress, which raises your stress hormones. Since stress hormones are tied to your being awake, this is bad news for sleep. Let's add to that that exercise raises your core body temperature. Again, not a bad thing. You're building up a sweat, so it's logical, right? However, your body wants a lower core temperature if you're to have optimal sleep.

Although you might feel that a tough evening workout helps you hit the pillow, the science says this is not in your best interests and, at a time when the odds are stacked against good sleep, my coaching would be to play the game and consider exercising earlier in the day. Yes, that kind of thing was OK when you were younger, but your hormones were also different back then.

So, if your schedule allows, exercising in the morning is best and, for rigorous exercise like HIIT, spinning, running, and so on, try not to work out after 4ish so that your stress hormones get a chance to come down alongside your core body temperature. This means you can tap into all the many benefits that come with moving your body without damaging the hormonal pattern your body craves. Now you just need to run the maths on when you are going to get that little breakfast in *before* you work out.

Like so many things to do with your health, consistency really matters. Getting exercise into your life regularly really helps your sleep. A huge amount of scientific work points to an interrelatedness between regular exercise and sleep, suggesting those who move their bodies consistently fall asleep faster, sleep longer with fewer wakings and enjoy a better quality of sleep.

Creating your sleep sanctuary

Remember the chemistry set that is your body? We're still doing that work. In chemical reactions, temperature is important, and that's the case here. If you've been through perimenopause, you'll know all about getting hot and bothered at night and the 'joy' that can bring.

Wearing lightweight bedclothes and choosing the right tog duvet can be one of a host of things that can help, but you should also consider room temperature. Even if you're a person who likes to stay warm, the best temperature for your room is between 15°C and 18°C.

You will want to do what you can to avoid having a high core body temperature because studies show people who struggle to sleep have higher core temperatures. So how can you do that?

We talked earlier about not exercising at night because this raises your core body temperature. You might try a bath. Taking a warm bath when you want to cool down sounds counterintuitive since a bath is going to raise your core body temperature.

But here's what happens (and this will allow you to play the game of hacking those sleep hormones): when you have a hot bath 90 minutes before bed, though you might feel you're getting hotter, the water stimulates your thermoregulatory system to push any 'hotness' from your core to your hands and feet, and this helps you fall asleep quicker.

If you've had children, you've probably seen first-hand the power of the bath for a good night's sleep. The evening routine of bath, story and bed is a winner. If you're doubting this could work for you, try it. Combine that bath with some nice, natural smellies and that's some of your evening self-care sorted if nothing else.

Since we're talking about temperature, every woman knows that it is impossible to get to sleep when you have cold feet. Simply, women are less good at warming their extremities than men, and this gets significantly worse if you're unfortunate enough to have an underactive thyroid. Don't forget the warm foot bath and/ or the snuggly socks if this is you.

We tend to stay up later than our ancestors because we can but going to bed after 11pm puts you at a hormonal disadvantage. Ideally, you want to get in as many sleep hours between 10pm and 2am, when melatonin is high and your sleep quality will be the very best. Getting the same number of hours sleep but going to bed far later isn't the same because you'll have missed too much of that extra-special quality sleep time. Nature is giving you the cues, so it's probably a good idea to start to follow them.

You can gently help your body to take advantage of this hormonal pattern by fixing your night-time lighting set-up. That's the business of dimming lights, getting an eye mask, maybe some blue light blocking glasses if you feel you need them - playing the game of hormones.

But, look, we all have our stuff we have to do and want to do, and no one would be able to do all of the things all of the time that would make a difference. Work out the aspect of your health that either bothers you most or you think might be easiest to start with and prioritise that one thing. Thoughts on how to do that towards the end of the book.

10-second recap

Light plays a big part in getting your body ready for sleep so dim lights in the evenings, put all screens in night shift mode after dark, and buy yourself a silk eye mask if you don't already have one. Minimise alcohol where you can as it's a big sleep-killer, and have a caffeine curfew after 2pm. Even if you reckon it has no effect on your sleep, it *will* be affecting the quality of your sleep.

CHAPTER 13
STRESS & YOUR METABOLISM

You may know a thing or two about how stress affects your own body. I am going to tell you about the science of it in a moment and, if you didn't already have an inkling, it's terrible news for your midlife metabolism - especially as a woman.

Here's an entirely made-up but pretty typical conversation I have with people about stress.

Me: I think stress could be a big factor for you.

You: No one died, I haven't just got divorced. I don't think I'm under a lot of stress.

Me: Even the relentlessness of daily living, going to work, and constantly feeding teenagers is enough in midlife. And traffic jams.

You: Everyone is stressed. There's literally nothing I can do about it. I can handle it.

Me: I really think the answer to what you want lies, at least in part, in dealing with the impact of stress.

You: Don't you know how busy I am? I don't have time for this unless you can prove this is definitely a thing or I literally fall down and am unable to carry on.

Testing your stress

Getting women to focus on stress management is a hard-sell unless you feel so awful you can't get out of bed or you're staring at test results that demonstrate your cortisol levels are off. You can do urine tests (DUTCH test) for metabolites of cortisol or saliva tests to spot whether your stress hormones are following the correct daily pattern. Some people are also genetically predisposed to make stress hormones more readily and clear them less well than others. This might be you if you're quick to feel the effects of stress and stay riled long after an argument has finished. In my practice we check this out with a DNA test (the nervous system one). And, if you've ever worn a continuous blood glucose monitor, you will probably have seen the following: on days when you do not sleep and/or are stressed, your blood glucose climbs much higher than on regular days. The stress doesn't have to be great. Have I already told you how my blood glucose spiked in a sad part in the *Eddie the Eagle* movie? So just imagine what *Toy Story 4* does to you!

These little stresses are part and parcel of life and do not need to be 'fixed'. What *is* a problem is how you feel and how your body behaves when it has been under *constant* pressure.

The point of testing is to give you conclusive proof there is something you must work on. In my experience, without the evidence in black and white, women typically won't take action in this area of life because it means either stopping doing some of the things they feel they *have to* do or else being asked to do extra things (like relaxing).

What stresses you out?

The stuff that puts stress on the body is called a 'stressor' and not all stressors are bad. In fact, it's not a goal to have no stress hormones in your body. This is a terrible thing since these hormones fulfil specific functions, like having higher cortisol in the morning to help you feel springy and ready for the day. So the problem is too much or too little and at the wrong time.

Stress can be a physical thing that happens to the body, an emotional or traumatic experience, or it can be imagined - you get a surge of stress hormones just by worrying about something like a big meeting coming up at work or something someone said that upset you. It can even be created as a result of the food, drinks or drugs (recreational or pharmaceutical) and even your environment.

The following is not an exhaustive list:

- Life events: grief/ sadness, change of circumstances (birth of a child, marriage, divorce, new cohabiting situation), unresolved trauma, PTSD, general anger (big and small, even traffic counts).
- Organisational: work pressures (losing a job, starting a new one), pressure (high-pressure work environment, pressure to pass exams), work deadlines, the relentless juggle of life, work and kids.
- Financial: bills, unexpected expenses, inflation/ cost of living.
- Social: conflict with others including relationship problems or toxic friends or family, bullying or abuse (online or real life).
- Physiological: injuries, accidents, pregnancy, past or current health conditions.
- Lifestyle: poor diet, undereating, overeating, too much fasting, food allergies and intolerances, not enough sleep, too much caffeine, too much alcohol, too much cardio like long runs, recreational or pharmaceutical drugs, lack of boundaries, watching the news, doing too many chores you hate.
- Environmental: bright lights, environmental chemicals, mould, dental amalgams, bacterial overgrowth in the gut, frequent flying, electromagnetic fields, noise, excess heat or cold, pollution, world events like war or natural disasters.
- Even winning the lottery!

Not everyone will feel stressed by the same things. For some, the small stuff is the big stuff, and that's OK. It comes down to your personal outlook and your level of resilience, and it's not for any of us to judge.

A couple of things I personally notice as far as stress in midlife goes: I cry a lot more now than I ever did, and I get annoyed by much smaller things than before. As a general note, "overwhelm" often features very high up on a list of complaints of women going through menopause and really this is caused by the loss of resilience.

If stress is so important for health, why don't the doctors do anything about it?

While there is a giant amount of scientific literature discussing the negative impact of stress on the human body, the modern medical model does not hold much truck with it because stress is not something doctors can fix with a pill. Most doctors are not geared up for dispensing lifestyle advice and their practices have no framework to support patients in following a lifestyle plan.

Why do we get stressed?

If too much stress is going to harm us, why do we get stressed? The human body hasn't evolved much since cavewoman days. The stress response at that time made logical sense.

In the days of caves, the stress involved whether we would get eaten by the sabre-tooth tiger before we got home safely from the hunt. In order to safely navigate our path home, the stress response would kick in. You might have heard people talk about the fight or flight response and this is it. Imagine how helpful the following would be if you needed to either run away from or hit said tiger with a big stick:

- Glucose is released from stores in the muscles to give you a burst of energy you can use to run fast.
- You breathe faster to take in more oxygen to make movement more powerful.
- Your heart beats faster to carry glucose and oxygen to the cells that require them to make energy.
- Your blood thickens to limit bleeding in case of injury.
- For the same reason, blood is diverted away from the surface of your skin, the digestive and reproductive systems (since digesting food and having babies ranks lower in priorities than staying alive).
- Your senses heighten and peripheral vision improves - superpowers in the making.
- Your brain is poised for split-second decisions but it's not that good at conscious decision making and logical thinking.
- Your palms and the soles of your feet become sweaty to improve traction for running or climbing.
- Cortisol is a powerful painkiller, so if you get injured, you're not going to know about it until later, enabling you to keep fighting life despite injury.

What's the problem with getting stressed?

From an evolutionary perspective, this stress mechanism was a winning formula but it was designed as a short and temporary measure. With the circumstances you find yourself in today, the mechanism works directly against your health and sets the stage for weight and metabolism problems. Today's stressors can be small but relentless or less frequent but very significant. Either way, they do not usually mean immediate physical danger and they are rarely something you can get on top of by running away or punching someone (and sometimes, more's the pity).

So you're not using the extra glucose or oxygen provided by the stress response. This means you're left with:

- Elevated glucose levels (leading to insulin resistance)
- Elevated oxygen levels (resulting in oxidation and inflammation)
- Thickened blood (an intro into cardiovascular disease and high blood pressure)
- Added to this, the digestion, reproduction, repair and maintenance functions get switched off. They're not needed for tiger-fighting even if that wasn't actually in your plans today. This creates the perfect backdrop for chronic illness, inflammation and weight gain.

Now you know all this, it's easy to see how something that seems minor at first glance – regular stress caused by too much work, not enough rest, poor diet, and anything else you care to tick off that list – could be messing with your health in different ways and different areas of your body.

How to know if you're stressed

There is no definitive list. You don't have to get tests run to decide you're experiencing the effects of stress. Everyone is stressed and, if you're wondering whether you're stressed enough, you probably are but here are some other signs your body is crying out for help:

1. You are constantly knackered - if fatigue is becoming a problem, it might actually be from any of the lifestyle, emotional or physical stress I listed earlier.
2. Your mood is unpredictable – when you have multiple reasons to be stressed out every day, you're probably focusing on your stressors more

than anything else. This causes overwhelm, panic, anxiety, and many more emotions that can lead to moodiness and agitation.
3. Your anxiety is getting worse - people with chronic stress find their anxiety is heightened, and those with anxiety find that stress affects them more readily. If you have an anxiety disorder, it is even more important for you to recognise the signs of stress and try to keep it under control as best you can.
4. You feel confused and lack focus – stress causes brain fog, which can lead to confusion, poor concentration, and that fuzzy feeling inside your head.
5. Other things to watch for include insomnia, lightheadedness on standing, menstrual irregularities, reduced immunity, reduced sex drive, craving for salty foods, digestive problems like IBS.

The straw that broke the camel's back

Being stress free is a pretty unrealistic goal. We all need a little external (and maybe internal) pressure from time to time to do our best giving a presentation or a speech, going to a big event, or acting in an am-dram play, for example. But we also need to ensure stress levels don't get too high. It's a balancing act, and I'm going to give you some ideas in the next chapter on how to get almost immediate traction without having to vastly change your life. Of course, you will need to do something different, but let's try not to make 'getting less stressed' stressful. And, remember, it's not about removing all stress… You can handle a lot but you cannot handle it all. When you try to handle it all, all of the time, it's not going to go so well. Ever heard of the straw that broke the camel's back? That.

The hormone that is even bigger than cortisol

Much of this metabolism business is about your hormones and it's useful to know there is a hierarchy of hormones. If there's one hormone more potent than cortisol, it's this: oxytocin.

Oxytocin

If you're come across oxytocin before, I'm betting it's because you had a baby.

Oxytocin plays a starring role in mums bonding with their baby. Oxytocin is often called the "love hormone". It's the neurotransmitter involved in initiating labour contractions, floods you with love for your newborn, and lets down (or 'ejects') milk during breastfeeding. It's also a feel-good neurotransmitter that helps build trust and creates emotional bonding. It also enhances empathy and makes you faithful. As a side note, it additionally improves glucose uptake in muscle (which is a good thing) as well as insulin sensitivity and reduces hunger. In the context of your midlife metabolism, one of the most valuable functions of oxytocin is its ability to counteract cortisol. So, oxytocin, welcome.

This amazing hormone acts as a natural antidote to stress. When oxytocin levels rise, they help offset the negative effects of cortisol, which as you already know, directly acts against every health goal you could have. So, a boost in oxytocin can create a more balanced chemical environment, which is especially crucial during midlife when your hormones are - sometimes literally - raging.

How to get more oxytocin

In all likelihood, your birthing years are over so where else can you get oxytocin? It's easier than you think - and you'll enjoy doing it!

- **Physical touch:** hugging, holding hands, massages, sex and masturbation.
- **Social connections:** spending time with loved ones. Social bonds are more critical than ever during midlife transitions.
- **Pet therapy:** cuddles with pets, especially dogs and cats. Yay!
- **Mindfulness and meditation:** mindfulness practices or meditation.
- **Listening to music:** music, especially when it evokes strong emotions. Singing and dancing along amplify the effect.
- **Helping others:** acts of kindness, including volunteering, gift-giving, or just assisting someone in need.

> **10-second recap**
>
> Stress is terrible news for your midlife metabolism and, from perimenopause onwards women are biologically less well able

to deal with it so you must create an action plan to dial down stress. If you know you have been dealing with a lot over the years and you're feeling exhausted, or you want to know how well genetically your body is likely to handle stress, ask me about testing. One way or another - even if you don't especially feel it - stress *will* be killing your health.

CHAPTER 14
CREATE AN ANTI-STRESS ACTION PLAN

It's beyond unhelpful for anyone to tell you to be less stressed. And yet here I am trying my own version of that so sorry and everything…My intention with this chapter is for you to spend a little time looking at the 'big picture' of your life and see if you can spot the low hanging fruit, which means to identify the stressors that are the easiest to get rid of and the situations that are simplest to fix. It's not often that we take the time to do this kind of review of our life and, in my view, it's probably an activity that's worth doing every few months: just checking in with how things are for you and what inputs you have in your life that aren't serving you.

Let me give you an example:

While quitting your stressful job is not necessarily going to be practical, these are some things that might be possible. Which are most relevant to you?

- Not getting enough sleep
- Not eating properly during the day
- Relying on tea and coffee to keep your energy levels up
- Eating at your desk or in the car
- Having a glass or two of wine every night
- Evening snacking
- Lots of evening screen time (blue light exposure) - late-night social media scrolling or decompressing late into the night with Netflix (dopamine at the wrong time)

Find your tipping point

You can probably think back to a time when you were 'on fire' with this whole eating and living well business. Not literally, obviously, but what I mean is that whatever you were doing just *worked* and everything went just as you wanted it to and felt easy.

And then, well, life started to take over, things slipped and slid and, before you knew it, you were back to eating crisps in the car.

It can feel hard to even see *how* you might get yourself back on track because the work to do seems so monumental.

The answer? Find your tipping point and take action right there.

What is a 'Tipping Point'?

In epidemiology, the tipping point is that moment when a small change tips the balance of a system and brings about a large change, as described by *New York Times* writer and author Malcom Gladwell. He's talking about big social change, of course. I'm talking about not secret-eating the biscuits.

Your tipping point is the thing that, if it goes right, everything else in life follows. You release a cascade of good habits through your life and soon whatever you're up to feels possible. But if it goes wrong, it knocks down all those good habits like dominoes. Since a lot of your habits may be increasing the total stress load on your body (chocolate biscuits, late nights, etc.), finding your personal tipping point is a worthwhile exercise.

What's to know about your tipping point is it's not set in stone. This week, the tipping point might be ensuring you get into bed to have enough of a stab at an eight-hour sleep stretch. Last month it might have been being firmer about work boundaries or saying 'no' more often to social engagements.

Given that it's easier to fix one thing rather than a whole load of stuff, get curious about what the *one* thing is that makes a real difference in your life. Really be in the enquiry here. If you could wave a magic wand in that area, what is the area you'd change?

When I'm working with clients, two things tend to come up with alarming frequency: planning and sleep.

Let's take the example of sleep as tipping point

If you make sleep your priority, getting more of it would immediately impact on your stress levels, you would awake more refreshed and have the time to get yourself a decent breakfast or lunch to take to work so you're not relying on Sandra's gifted Devon fudge or the birthday doughnuts. You'd also be less likely to have to prop up your energy levels with too many teas and coffees, which might impact on the upcoming night's sleep. By sleeping more, eating a better breakfast and lunch, you'll likely avoid eating a mini meal as you prep the dinner, and maybe won't snack after your dinner either.

We'll talk more about this in the final part of the book, but it all comes down to making something a priority; making it an actual project. I suspect part of the reason you don't do the stuff you say you want to do is that you *could* make a start at any time it took your fancy. And because you *could* do the thing at any time, it floats around without a start point, yes?

Do more of what you love, and less of what you hate

This sounds obvious but stay with me. My practical experience of working with clients on their wellbeing tells me this: astonishingly few women are really clear on the *specific* things that fill them with joy and the *specific* things they hate. Many people are resigned to things being 'the way it is'. Some things are fixed but there might be more that can be tweaked than you think so don't write your life off as 'it's just like this'.

Women rarely prioritise their own non-work and non-caring (for children, parents, pets) responsibilities. Sweeping generalisation, but the women I meet are used to putting their own needs after everyone else's and, by the time they get to the menopause years, this plan has backfired and they need to retrain themselves by focussing on their own self-care.

Let's have a look at the low-hanging fruit; the stuff you can lose or change without too much bother…

Every day, there will be a bunch of activities, tasks and habits. There will be those that interest you or that you love, those that bore or frustrate you, or that you hate but 'have' to do. The first task is to work out which they are. Few people take the time to be specific and the thing you like or don't like will often lie less in the act but more in the *detail* like timing or other circumstances.

The reason why the exercise that follows is a good idea is because it helps create balance and reduce stress, and we both know that would be a good thing right now. And how can you reduce stress? Do less stuff that stresses you and more stuff that fills you with joy, therefore acting as a counterbalance, a bit like an old-fashioned set of scales. On one side you have activities that restore you and, on the other, those that challenge you. You don't have to change *everything* overnight but you will have the raw data to think on and choose what you want to put on the table.

Recreating balance exercise

Find a quiet time and a quiet enough space to do this exercise. Don't worry, there aren't many questions but they are important. If you need to pop on some noise cancelling headphones to zone out other people, do that. I want you to write down your answers rather than keep them in your head. It's too much to remember, why put that extra stress on yourself? That can be either the notes section of your phone or tablet, or a journal or notebook. Take a page for each question. Don't overthink it. Get as much down as you can and don't worry if some of the ideas overlap. There isn't a correct answer, it's just what you feel.

1. I feel my best when I am …

    Examples: sleeping well, exercising daily, on point with my food, making time to see friends and family, getting up and moving about rather than sitting at my desk for too long.

2. I feel low in energy, overwhelmed, resentful, anxious or worried when I …

    Examples: have a poor night's sleep, say yes to too many things and have too much to do in a day, have to do the home admin, don't take a break at work, eat too much junk, spend too much time scrolling on social media.

3. I feel calm and peaceful when I …

    Examples: go out for a walk, read a good book, sit for a moment to just 'be', spend time colouring, crafting or being creative, listen to my favourite music.

4. I feel excited, empowered, or inspired when I …

    Examples: make time to exercise, regularly meet up with friends, go to the theatre, galleries, gigs or other creative events, attend a course/ seminar/ talk.

Now review what you have written, taking special note of question two since this is where the less good stuff is lurking. How much of your time do you spend doing the things that drain you? Is there anything that might counterbalance these depleting activities? If you notice you feel overwhelmed by the weekly shop, is it possible to go online? If you're frustrated by home admin, can tasks be shared among the family? Can you choose to be OK with some things the way they are and the way they aren't?

A side thought on delegating

Every woman I know feels - to some extent or another - they are doing *everything* and no one is grateful. The only answer is not to do as much stuff. This is all at once simple and highly effective but it also requires a mindset shift. Because you need the control. That's right, only *you* know how the dishwasher needs to be loaded. Only you put everything back in the proper place. If you could teach yourself to delegate more, things would - over time - improve and you would feel less put upon. Changing things can feel impossible. Rome wasn't built in a day and, if you do nothing, nothing changes so here's something to just be with for a while and try out at your leisure.

Next time you are fuming about tasks akin to the dishwasher business, ask yourself, 'What would happen if I didn't load the dishwasher?' Then 'What is the worst that could happen if I didn't load the dishwasher?'. Some of the stuff ends up in the wrong place? I get that; it's annoying but nobody ever died from finding the Pyrex badly filed.

So now we've cleared that up, as long as there is no real prospect of someone getting physically hurt or financially disadvantaged, and it's not going to be emotionally damaging for you, you could just *not do something*. Think of all that time you would save if you didn't have to load the dishwasher and you gave yourself the permission for it to be OK if things weren't always the way you wanted them. Think of all that time adding up through the week…

And what if you could off-load something else: kids getting all their stuff out for school (if they're still young); children (or partners) loading and emptying the washing machine, re-enforcing the rule that everyone has their own set of jobs in the house, or whatever is a good fit for you.

Spend more time doing things you love

Now look at the remainder of the questions you answered above. How much time do you spend on the restoring, nourishing activities? They don't have to be fancy or time consuming. The activities could be as simple as reading a book or taking time to do your nails. I've always been an avid reader, for example, and this year have made a valiant effort. I always have a real book on the go; I have the Kindle app with another book on my phone (because you never know when opportunity may strike); and I listen to audiobooks when I walk or drive.

Imagine the 'nourishing activities' that fill your cup of joy were on sticky notes and you have your diary in front of you. Where could they slot in? There is always more time than you think.

"Self-care isn't selfish"

I had to put that bit in quotes because, well, it's a bit cheesy. But it is true and it's one of the things that I find myself talking to nearly all my clients about. In the very broadest sense, self-care is what is at the opposite end of the spectrum to health care, where you might seek professional help for long-term or acute conditions or major trauma. Edging nearer to 'self-care', you have things like managing your own minor ailments like colds and flu and even brushing your teeth. But self-care in the sense I mean it now is replenishing your spirit by taking care of your own happiness and doing little things *every day* just for the joy of doing it.

Sometimes when I start on this with clients, there are a few eye rolls. This is so essential for women as we get older because of all the stuff about declining lady hormones and stress, and this is why I created a programme called The Self-Care Fix.

Self-care is the recognition that only you can make yourself happy (although other people can obviously contribute to it) and that, if you make sure that you dedicate some time every day purely for your own enjoyment, you will have more fun, you will be more fun to be around, and you will have far greater reserves to deal with the stresses of everyday life.

Self-care is a skill and it is a discipline. It is something that can be very easy to do (which is why it is something we often don't bother to do).

So, this week I invite you to make a list of at least 20 things (even really frivolous things) that you love to do just because they make you happy or they delight you. Just so you know, housework will never be self-care, however much you like a nicely pressed sheet. It needs to be an actual list - either in a journal or in the notes section of your phone or tablet - because when you most need a little self-care, you are often not in a resourceful state of mind. If you've had a crappy day for whatever reason, you won't have the wherewithal to scroll through the Rollerdex of your mind for things you could do to make you feel better.

You don't have to spend long for this to be effective. Some snippets from my self-care list if you need some inspiration: taking a lovely hot bath, sitting in the sunshine, reading a few chapters from a good thriller, watching my favourite comedy show, singing along to my favourite songs on Magic at the Musicals on the radio, or catching up with a friend. The important thing is these are all things that feel good *in the moment*. Although exercise is also important for your midlife metabolism, it is not self-care. It fits into the movement category, and we'll be talking more about that in the next chapter.

A side note on time

"But I don't have the time," you might be saying to yourself. In reality, when you make some extra time for *you*, suddenly more time appears in the day as if by magic, which I can only explain by way of saying that, when you focus on your own happiness as well as your job, your family and so on, you will have a much more positive, can-do attitude that gets things done more efficiently.

If you're still in the 'yes, but…' camp, we'll come back to it. In the last part of this book, which is all about putting the science into your actual life, we'll be taking a look at how you are spending your time. There might be a little more spare time than you think; perhaps not giant swathes but enough to do something good and feel the benefit.

So, just for the fun of it right now and without being concerned with how you will do any of this, complete the exercise about what fulfils you and also draw up that self-care list.

I hope this doesn't come across as a chore. Self-care is - by its very nature - enjoyable. It helps cheer you up or pull you out of a hole if you've been having an emotionally tricky day. Which leads me nicely onto my final point before I rest my case for self-care: self-care is one of the best fixes for emotional eating.

Stop eating your feelings

We don't always eat because we are hungry. We eat because we can and maybe because we're not sure when we'll have another chance to, because we need comfort or we're celebrating. Or commiserating. We eat because we're bored. This is called non-hunger eating. Literally, eating when you are not hungry. Part of that is emotional eating; eating in response to a specific emotion you are feeling.

Most people will at some stage have eaten when they feel a bit low. In a world in which we are often surrounded by food, eating can be a common response. There's nothing inherently wrong with emotional eating. But when *sometimes* becomes *a lot of the time*, you might be slipping into disordered eating, which is the term used to describe irregular eating patterns rather than a diagnosis and is not the same as having an eating disorder.

I'm not going to go down the road of emotional eating too - that's a whole other story - but suffice to say there can be some very deep-rooted reasons why people overeat, many of these entrenched in the past and related to finding a substitute for love, belonging, grief, bullying, protection and self-sabotage. I think it's a good idea to seek help for this if this is more than an occasional problem. If it's a now-and-again thing, these two things will help:

- Self-care to fill up your little cup of joy, while simultaneously making you more resilient.
- Mindful eating, which we discussed in the chapter *How To Eat*, which helps bring greater awareness to eating through one mindful meal.

A further reason why you should definitely focus on self-care is that it's far better to replace *eating* something 'nice' with *doing* something nice for yourself.

We are so time-poor that rewarding ourselves with 'treat' foods like cake and biscuits is the easiest way to show ourselves we care. In my experience, so little of why you eat what you eat has to do with nourishing your body. The far greater part is to do with how you feel about yourself and about life in general. Eating half a packet of chocolate biscuits is much easier than figuring out – not to mention getting – what you really need, which might be a way to de-stress, feel loved, get attention, kick back your heels, or even sleep. Most people are almost completely out of touch with their own bodies.

When I'm working with clients, we focus a great deal on lifestyle and mindset because it is a critical factor in deciding whether you make healthy food choices. Simple fact: if you feel stressed or miserable, the chocolate biscuits are always going to win – unless you have a plan in place for dealing with those things.

Guided meditation & stress relief

Meditation is the art of focussing your mind on one thing. It's been around for millennia but really started being studied for its health benefits in the 1970s. Now, thanks to a lot of phone apps, mediation is mainstream, and specifically the approachable sort called guided meditation.

There are many reasons to try guided meditation, all backed by science, including relief from stress and anxiety, improving emotional wellbeing, enhancing self-awareness, controlling pain, and improving sleep. It is even now being studied for its ability to reduce menopausal symptoms.

Guided meditation is like the lazy girl's meditation. It's literally someone guiding you through what to do so there is no getting it wrong. And you are reminded to gently bring your train of thought back to the task at hand when your mind inevitably starts wandering to your to-do list and whatever else is in your brain at the time. There is no expectation that you must be 'good' and that your mind should not wander. Quite simply, it is the most effective and certainly the quickest intervention I know for helping you empty your head and release stress.

Since guided meditation is about keeping you in the here and now, doing more of that is enormously beneficial for nixing the over-analysing we do about our lives, the situations and people in it. When you focus on the present, your anxiety will naturally lower as this is often based on overthinking what has already happened that cannot be changed or that which hasn't and might not actually happen.

This is a simplification, of course. In perimenopause, a lot can happen in the arena of anxiety and, if you have a thyroid problem, this can multiply. I've seen first-hand time and again, these ten-minute guided exercises are the gold. Everyone can afford ten minutes for the benefits it brings.

> **Katie's story**
>
> 'It's taken a while but now I can honestly say guided meditation is part of my routine and I love it because it makes me calmer and more together. I don't do it every single day but most days and I miss it when I don't. It took a while to work out whether it was better for me to do it after I dropped my kids off at school or at night. I was hit and miss for a bit but I've now worked out that the best time for me is before bed.
>
> Then I also have the benefit that I am calm right before I go to sleep.'

> **10-second recap**
>
> The number one thing to do to dial down your stress is to work out your tipping point and, instead of focussing on all the things you could be doing, to get this one thing nailed and the ripples will spread to other areas of your life. After that, consider taking on one of the other sure-fire ways to feel calmer: getting clear on what lights you up and drains you about your life, filling your happiness cup with self-care and dedicating 10 minutes a day to guided meditation. Which will you start with?

CHAPTER 15
THE RIGHT EXERCISE

There are plenty of people who absolutely love exercise and really this is your goal: to find a way you love to move that also brings the results that you want. For many - myself included - exercise often only features because we want to keep our weight in check and, if we could get a bit of sexy muscle definition that helped us ditch the bingo wings and look good in short-sleeved tops, well, that would be exciting beyond reason.

Come closer. I have news.

Movement and exercise are two equally important elements in improving your metabolic health. They are two slightly different things. For the purposes of this book, movement means all types of movement that is not traditional 'exercise'. That might mean standing at a desk rather than sitting, walking up the stairs rather than taking the lift, and generally 'being more active'.

Exercise, well, I think we both know what we're talking about here but what often surprises the women who come to work with me is that not all exercise is created equal and that the 'best' exercise in midlife does not involve running. We'll come onto how to get more movement into your life in the next chapter but here, just let's talk about exercise more conceptually right now.

All kinds of movement are good for you. I'm sure you heard the evidence for exercise, which is enormous and ranges from boosting your mood to helping you sleep better. But exercise will not necessarily help you lose weight, and that goes for all women and not just menopausal women like us.

Mic drop.

Exercise does not help you lose weight

Research over the last handful of decades that has tracked exercise levels and obesity rates shows that, despite people in the developed world engaging in more exercise activities, obesity rates did not fall as everyone thought they would. They have, in fact, increased, and this tells us that something else and not exercise is behind the problem. Diet and exercise are important but not equally so. In this book *The Obesity Code*, Jason Fung puts it brilliantly like this: 'Diet is Batman, exercise is Robin. Diet does 95% of the work and deserves all the attention… Exercise is like brushing your teeth. It is good for you and should be done every day. Just don't expect to lose weight'. He's not a whack job, he has the science on this and is a preeminent doctor in the field of obesity and diabetes, so we should listen up.

I know you have deeply ingrained in your mind that in order to lose weight you need to eat less and move more but here's what typically happens when you go down that path.

Aside from your body adjusting to the lower number of calories you are eating, becoming more efficient and so you burn fewer calories each day while doing the same work, if you're not eating enough, you will start to lose muscle mass. When you lose lean muscle, your metabolic rate (the speed at which everything works) drops too, and this means your body needs even less fuel to power you through the day. It's a vicious circle, and this is why so many women who go on the 'eat less, move more' diet end up in a world of emotional pain where they are hungry, sluggish and, when they go back to their regular eating habits, put all the weight back on (and often more).

You might already have experienced one of the problems with the 'eat less, move more' situation and that is, when you move more, you also feel hungrier and, when you combine this with a calorie deficit, trouble is afoot.

According to a 2009 study, the "hunger hormone" ghrelin spikes after a workout in women, while leptin, which tells the brain that you're full, plummets. Not so in men. So after a workout, women tend to eat more, which puts them at risk of gaining weight – the exact opposite of what most women are trying to achieve.

Men don't experience this same hormonal fluctuation. Researchers are not sure why that is. They can only speculate, and one theory is that it's the female body's way to avoid energy deficits to preserve fertility and perpetuate the species. In the female body, a lack of calories suppresses ovulation and hormones that make reproduction possible.

And, since you did that workout, you may also feel you have 'earned' the right to eat. Overcompensating is very real. And there's more. When you move more, you will be more inclined to rest on your laurels doing less for the remainder of the day so your non-exercise activity is reduced.

I'm not saying don't exercise. Far from it. As midlife women we must do the work to shore up muscle and keep us strong and bendy for life - just choose the *right* exercise.

Dieters are more likely to choose cardio over strength and this is a mistake

The eat less, move more diets typically advocate the type of exercise that burns more calories since they assert it's all about creating a calorie deficit. That means, when you follow this religion you must pick high intensity exercise like running, spin classes and the like. There's nothing inherently wrong with this type of exercise so no need to panic if you love working out like this. But, remember, exercise is a stressor on the body so this kind of high intensity exercise - when done regularly - can create too much stress and this goes directly against most women's goals for doing it in the first place.

Frequent high intensity exercise also signals to your body that you want endurance and not strength, so your body prioritises losing weight from your muscles (which are not needed for endurance) and this further lowers your metabolic rate. To top it all, you'll begin storing more energy in your fat cells - literally packing those out preferentially over muscle as this is more convenient to access when you're doing long-haul cardio.

That is not to say you should not do any cardio. Different types of exercise are good for different things. Cardiovascular fitness is important for health but, if fat-loss is on your mind or you want to fix your midlife metabolism, you will not get there by doing this kind of workout. Cardio will burn more calories when you are actually exercising but, since you spend the majority of your day not exercising, it's far better to work on increasing your muscle mass so you can burn more calories (and improve your metabolism) when you are at rest.

> **Caron's story**
> Caron had been doing all the expected things she thought she should do to lose weight, including dropping her calories by 500 a day and doing five cardio sessions a week, including running and spin. She was used to years of punishing her body like this and was frustrated this approach was no longer keeping her weight in check.
>
> She wasn't sure how to square it with her brain that she was being asked to eat more food and switch out some of her cardio for strength training. Even when she started noticing the results, she couldn't quite believe it was true.
>
> 'It feels like I am somehow cheating the system,' she told me.

Burning more energy without lifting a finger

Most people think of their energy expenditure in relation to the time spent 'burning calories' by exercising but this only accounts for 5-10% of the energy you use in a day. It's called exercise activity thermogenesis or EAT. Know of a local pub quiz? Book yourself in now! The remaining energy is used when you process your food (the thermal effect of food or TEF), which accounts for another 5-10%; or through other kinds of movement that aren't categorised as exercise like walking about and generally living your life (this is non-exercise activity thermogenesis or NEAT), and that makes up 15-25% of total energy expenditure. We'll talk more about how to increase that in the next chapter. The greatest energy expenditure through the day is your basal metabolic rate or BMR, which is how much energy your body expends just by existing. That makes up a whopping 55-75% and you use this energy even when you're asleep or bingeing on your favourite Netflix series. Since muscle uses up more energy to maintain, you will increase your basal metabolic rate by building more muscle.

You must lift weight

You might need a little mindset tweak for this part. I want you to put out of your mind some massive Arnold Schwarzenegger bodybuilder guy when I say this, but to get healthy, lose weight and boost your metabolism in midlife you need muscle. For most women reading this book, that means building more muscle. Don't let your mind stray to the fact that muscle weighs more than fat and/ or, if you weigh more you will be bigger. You could be the same weight as you are now and look amazing as a trim and toned version of yourself with more muscle, or stay a couple of dress sizes larger, with more fat and looking frumpier. Same weight, but how you feel about yourself when you look in the mirror will be very different. The scale does not discriminate, which is one of the great many reasons it is an imperfect way to measure your health. There are a gazillion reasons why building muscle is good for you but no more so than for your metabolic health.

Obviously, you already have *some* muscle otherwise your body wouldn't be able to move or function. When people talk about 'muscle' they are usually referring to skeletal muscle and this helps with mobility, balance and strength - all things we lose as we get older. Having strong muscles is a sign of good physical function.

The problem is, you're gradually losing muscle all the time. You'll lose 2% between 35 and 55, a further 2% in the next two decades, and the downhill slide continues after that. It may not sound a great deal, but it is. As you get older, you lose muscle. It's even got a name - sarcopenia - and the decline starts at 30 and you'll lose 3-5% every decade. It's not in your interest to lose muscle. People who have low skeletal muscle are also likely dealing with some of this, and I don't want that for you:

- Metabolic syndrome
- Obesity
- Diabetes
- Osteoporosis
- Struggle doing daily tasks
- Earlier death

Your muscles are glucose sponges

Let's do a bit of a recap: when you eat, the sugar (and anything that gets broken down into glucose) hits your bloodstream. Your muscles absorb any glucose they can, a bit like a sponge. If you only have a small amount of muscle, there's only so much they can soak up. Or maybe the sponge is full because you're not exercising enough for the contents to get wrung out. Either way, excess glucose stays in the bloodstream and that's not a good thing.

If your muscles are bigger (and that doesn't mean bulgy like a bodybuilder) and the sponge gets frequently wrung out, you can soak up more glucose, so there's less in the blood, you get fewer glucose spikes, less insulin is made, and there's less need to store the excess in the liver or your fat cells.

As an aside, the liver is also a bit like a sponge. Like your muscles, it can only store so much. You can't make it bigger but you can ensure it doesn't get over-full (non-alcoholic fatty liver disease) by 'wringing it out' - by taking a break from not eating (fasting).

The added benefit for women who lift is they also experience fewer hot flushes - by up to 44%, and this happens because you are improving your vascular health, which then has a knock-on effect on temperature regulation in the body.

How to get more muscle

- Do bodyweight exercises like pushups, tricep dips, squats
- Use a resistance band
- Lift dumbbells - even soup cans work if you're very new to this
- Use weight machines (or free weights) in the gym
- Do pilates (but you can't *only* do pilates to gain the muscle you need)

I'm not the best person to advise on this but you'll find plenty of people online with advice for strength training specifically for menopausal women. The exercise folk you'll meet online likely won't be qualified enough to dispense *personalised* nutrition and lifestyle advice but soak up all the muscle training info you need from them.

Just like personalised nutrition, if the budget is there for one-to-one fitness, do that. A personal trainer will be able to craft a progressive programme that challenges you while at the same time takes into consideration any injuries and other personal circumstances that might otherwise hinder your progress.

If you've not done the strength training thing before, start with two or three 30-60-minute workouts a week at times that best suit your schedule. If you're a member of a gym, the trainers are often super helpful, especially for newbies who might one day end up being their private clients. If you're having a go at home, how you get started depends very much on what kind of equipment - if any - you have available.

Some thoughts:

If the weights you have at home belong to someone who lifts heavier than you, don't start here. No one wants an injury right out of the blocks. You're probably better to get started with bodyweight or resistance bands (less than £10 online).

Google resistance workouts or at-home strength workouts for women over 40. Don't worry about your current abilities or lack thereof.

It's not a competition but if it were, it would be with yourself. Over time you will get better.

What if I can't work out?

There will almost always be something you can do. At 51, I was in better shape than I'd been in years in spite of a very slow healing ankle ligament problem and a dodgy shoulder.

Instead of using what you *can't* do as an excuse not to do anything, work out what you *can* do. If you need some personal input but cannot afford a regular personal trainer on a regular basis, see if someone will do a one-off session or ad-hoc sessions to help you figure out what you can do with your current mobility or fitness level, and what is possible for you in your actual life. My first meeting with a personal trainer began with my announcing the reasons I couldn't work with her on a weekly basis followed by a long list of all my ailments and injuries.

Whatever you can or cannot do in the world of exercise, you can focus on the other work we talked about - eating, sleeping, and stress management.

Feeding your muscles

When you want to grow strong and build muscle, you need to fuel your muscles properly. This is called activating muscle protein synthesis. You don't need to turn into one of those muscle fanatics who meal-preps 20 chicken breasts for snacks but you must include enough protein in your diet. We talked about the importance of protein in an earlier chapter. You don't need to go mad but you do need to ensure you have protein at every meal, and also in any snacks you have.

> **10-second recap**
> Although it might feel that doing more of the kind of exercise that burns the most calories (like running and spin classes) is the way to lose weight, it will work against your midlife metabolism. Cardio should form part of an exercise regime to stay healthy more generally but if you want to lose weight and rev up your metabolism you need to build muscle. You won't get big unless you really, really go for it but you do need to stop the downhill slide of muscle wasting.

CHAPTER 16
GETTING A BIT MORE ACTIVE

A workout is only a small piece of the movement puzzle each day. Aside from your BMR (basal metabolic rate), which is the amount of energy you use up just by being alive, non-exercise movement (NEAT or non-exercise thermogenesis) makes up a big share of the energy you use up each day. This is all the other kinds of movement you do, from walking up the stairs to fidgeting, so it makes sense to do more of this if you can. This kind of movement doesn't increase your appetite like a proper workout can and, in case you were thinking you'll just do more of this type of movement to burn energy, don't forget that burning calories is not everything. You'll still need to build muscle to increase your basal metabolic rate, so you'll burn more energy while you rest, and because it improves your blood glucose control. This is why 'eat less, move more' is a huge over-simplification.

Having repeatedly said throughout the book that calories aren't everything, they are *something* and they do matter. The most important thing for your long-term health and your midlife metabolism is you get back in control of your blood glucose and insulin levels. Taking care you are not undereating and mucking up that aspect of metabolism, you need to ensure you use enough calories during the day to reach your happy weight. It is a very delicate balance - but one not won by rigorous calorie counting. An easy way to do this is by adding a little extra unstructured movement every single day, which over the course of the year can add up to pounds lost without breaking a sweat.

But I go to the gym...

Even if you are a regular gym-goer, it's still easy to live a sedentary life where you're sitting or lying down for the vast majority of it. Sedentary lifestyles negatively affect every aspect of health and the two main problems are that you burn less energy and you get stuck in one position for prolonged periods. It doesn't matter whether you have a fancy desk chair, one of those seated balls at your desk, an ergonomic kneeling chair or even no chair at all because you're using a standing desk. If you're in the same position for much of the day, it is not going to go well for you.

There's a lot of research into this NEAT business as a way of losing weight without having to become a gym bunny or otherwise work out how to fit more exercise into your already-overstuffed life. You've probably read magazine articles suggesting you get off the bus one stop earlier or park further away from work. It's that kind of thing. It's also ironing, squatting to pick up a box, cleaning, gardening, walking up and down stairs, walking the dog, standing up.

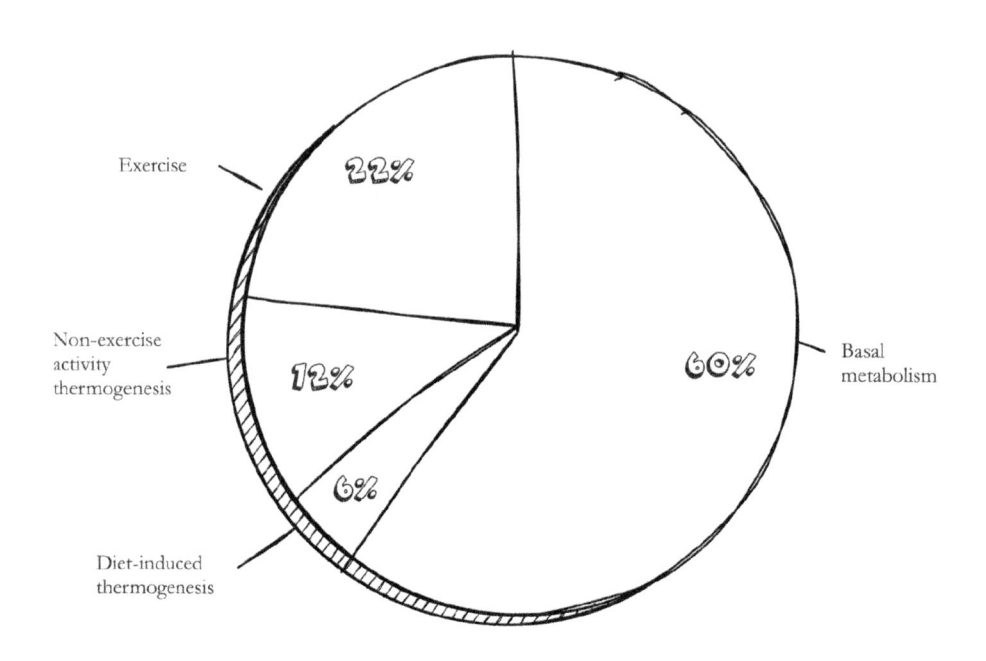

Exercise 22%
Non-exercise activity thermogenesis 12%
Diet-induced thermogenesis 6%
Basal metabolism 60%

How to dial up NEAT

When you're busy, it's easy to lose that zoomed-out overview of what you actually do in a day and be a bit fuzzy about how much movement goes on. This is completely normal but if you could be just a teeny bit more intentional about movement, your body and health would love you for it.

My advice is this: use a time planner (see the Resources section at the end of the book) to fill in your daily activities in detail, ideally as they happen. This should include everything, from waking up, sitting in bed drinking tea, getting ready for work, travelling to work. Get it all down. Often my clients are surprised by how much of the time they spend sitting down.

The second part of the job is to think creatively about what you could tweak so less of that time is spent on your bum.

Thoughts:
- Get a standing desk platform you can pop on top of your home desk - or ask your employer whether there's a budget for you to have one.
- You don't have to use the standing desk all day. In fact, my smartwatch assumes I'm sitting down if I stand at my desk too long and gives me the message, 'time to stand'. Alternate between standing up and sitting down. Aim for 50% standing.
- Mix up work activities so you're not sitting for long stretches.
- Take regular breaks away from your desk. Get up, stretch, walk about a bit. Stand up and maybe even walk about when on the phone (speaking or texting).
- Take the long way around to the kitchen/ bathroom.
- Walk to your colleague's desk (where practical) rather than phone or email them.
- If you work from home, can you vary how you sit? Spend some time sitting at your desk, some seated time cross legged on the floor, and so on. Before you start rolling your eyes, this is not supposed to be definitive - see what works for you. My office desk is a kneeling desk and I also sometimes use the kitchen table, which means my body is organised in a slightly different position. And I sometimes sit on the floor. It's rare but it occasionally happens.

That's just the work day.

Is there scope for an early morning walk (double benefit of getting the morning sunlight into your eyes, which is amazing for the nervous system, especially if you are stressed or struggle to sleep, as discussed elsewhere in the book)? Even 5-10 minutes works.

Or maybe a lunchtime or after-dinner walk. Both are helpful for digestion and avoiding blood glucose spikes.

If your children play sport, pace the sidelines or walk around the pitch for some of the time. Take the stairs more often than you take the lift.

Have a little jiggle in the kitchen to your favourite music as you do the washing up or load the dishwasher.

Do more gardening.

Get in random movement - calf raises or a few squats while you clean your teeth.

Try some mini walks. Longer walks are great but can be difficult to weave into your day. A five-minute walk around the block between work tasks is more do-able.

You get the drift. Your task is not to do *all* the things but try on a couple and see how they feel. Consistency is key. Like most things, when you do something often it becomes your normal.

Important notes about NEAT

Getting more NEAT doesn't have to be planned. You can go with the flow and simply choose to move a little more when the opportunity presents itself.

Don't start looking for the best NEAT to do. It's all good. Don't measure it, just be aware of doing more of it.

Enrol others in doing it too, whether that means having a family challenge or roping in a friend so you can keep each other accountable.

Getting your steps in

Many of my clients measure their steps. The goal many set for themselves is 10,000, a number entrenched in our public consciousness.

Fun fact, this came from a marketing campaign for a pedometer brand called Manpo-kei (which literally means 10,000 steps in Japanese) that was launched to get Japan fitter ahead of the 1964 Olympics in Tokyo. It wasn't based on any actual science at the time but was an arbitrary figure that sounded indicative of a healthy lifestyle. There's still not a lot of evidence that shows this specific number is magic but what we do know is that sedentary lifestyles are bad news for health and that moving more is helpful but that even as little as 6,000-8,000 might be enough to ward off chronic disease.

So what's my point?

A step counter like a smartwatch can help gauge how active you are. It's not the be-all and end-all but you can look back on your day with a measure of objectivity. Don't let that number intimidate you. Your job is not to be the best, it is to be better than yesterday. So if you only hit 2,000 steps yesterday, can you try for 3,000 today? 3,000 is not the end goal, but the point to note is actually setting a goal is helpful and not setting the bar ridiculously high is more likely to end in success.

Habit stacking

There are plenty of books that celebrate adding one activity you want to become a habit onto something you are already doing. This is called 'habit stacking' and the theory is that, because you are already successfully doing the one thing, you will continue to do it and you will also likely do the new thing without too much additional effort. This additional effort is called resistance and the thing that usually stops us doing new things is because they feel hard.

Think creatively about which habits you can stack together. If you already have a mindful morning routine (if not, try it out) that includes guided meditation, try adding a simple stretching routine. Five minutes is all you need to stay nimble.

If there are certain nights you're always watching the TV for a particular show, can you bring the ironing board in and, instead of sitting down to watch, stand to iron (two birds, one stone and all that).

Movement after meals

Your muscles are glucose sponges and building muscle by lifting weights (even your own bodyweight) is a great idea. Any kind of movement can be helpful for blood glucose control. This is how it works.

When you eat, the body breaks down the food into the units it can use - sugars (glucose) from the carbohydrate element, amino acids from the protein element and fatty acids from the fat. It takes a while for all this to happen inside your body, and your glucose levels will hit their peak within 90 minutes.

If you're already using up some of that glucose, you'll experience less of a spike. I'm hoping you are going to do the food work and, therefore, not be having a spike but this is exactly why a leisurely post Sunday lunch bike ride or walk is a good idea. By moving your body, you're using up the glucose as it hits your bloodstream meaning less glucose gets stored.

> **10-second recap**
> The amount of energy you use during exercise classes or going on a run is only a small percentage of the total energy you'll expend during a day. Every little bit of extra movement helps, whether it's alternating standing at your desk or sitting, pacing around at kids' sports matches or when you're on the phone, dancing in the kitchen or taking short walks around the block to clear your head. Your metabolism - and your waistline - will thank you for every last bit.

PART FOUR

CHAPTER 17
GET YOUR HEAD IN THE GAME

If enough were riding on it or if your life depended on it, I'll bet you know enough to do this all on your own and get a really great result that would change your life. The problem that most people have is doing everything consistently enough to get the results they want.

I don't say this to judge you because I was - and I still sometimes am - the same. Where there is not enough pain, where there isn't enough at stake to get you off the starting blocks and moving forward at pace, you will just do what you have always done. You will start, then you will stall, then you will probably berate yourself for your lack of consistent action. It's human nature.

When I'm creating a programme for clients, it's important for me to design their programme not only with their specific goals in mind but also with an understanding of why they want the transformation they want. For you, knowing your *why* is the key. You might have heard people talk about that before and think it's all a bit woo woo but the reason it matters is that to do anything consistently enough to get a result, you don't need *more knowledge* but more action. No one takes action unless they're clear about 'what's in it for me?'

Just wishing things were different is not enough. That's not very powerful. And is certainly not going to keep you going beyond next Friday. So ask yourself, what is the real motivation behind wanting to lose weight or eating more healthily? When you're filled with motivation, you'll find it easier to move rapidly towards your goal, and if you can harness that feeling, as well as the 'why', you will be able to stay on track when other attempts to sort out your weight or any other aspect of your health have failed.

If you've tried this already and your enthusiasm ended up waning, you're probably missing the step that comes *after* this step so stay with me for a moment.

Start by setting goals

How often do you reach your goals? If the answer is 'not very often', you may need to revisit your goal-setting strategy.

I'd like you to take a bit of time to think about what it is you'd like to change and why. I'm guessing one thing is losing a certain amount of weight but what else? Those irritating hot flushes? The lack of sleep? What is your goal *specifically*? Start with that. 'Get healthy' isn't a goal because it isn't specific. Neither is 'lose weight' but a specific (and realistic) amount is. Or it might be fitting into a specific outfit. Unless you are really clear what the scope of work actually is, it will be impossible to know that you have reached your goal.

The 'best' kind of goals are what's known as SMART goals, which means they are specific, measurable, achievable, realistic and time-bound.

Let's look at what that means in real life:

Specific. What do you actually want *specifically* and without being vague. Oftentimes, I find people err on the side of caution because of what others might think or concerns about what happens if they miss the mark. *Exercise: write down what you want, whether that's in a journal or in the notes section of your phone. This is important so don't skip this step because it makes it real.*

Measurable. How will you measure progress towards your goal? The number on the scale or (better still) the tape measure is a good guide for weight but if you are looking for improvement in hot flushes, digestive problems and so on, you'll need a way of measuring how things are for you right now. Use a basic scoring system. As long as you're consistent, it doesn't really matter what scale you use. I use a scale of 1-6 with clients. A score of one would be a low rating - the symptom really doesn't bother you at all. A six is something that is significantly impacting your life or it's as bad as it's ever been for you. You could measure as many symptoms as you like but I would choose no more than about three or four to keep track of.

Achievable. Give yourself a reality check. There's a balance between setting goals that are so easy they don't actually inspire you to do anything at all and those that, on reflection, might seem out of reach. There is a sweet spot between goals that feel a bit of a stretch and those that are over-optimistic or that require time you just don't have.

At the risk of sounding like a cheesy motivational quote, the magic really does exist outside of your comfort zone. So, aim for the stars rather than one of the planets farthest from the earth.

Relevant. Just check in with the goals you have written down. Are they really aligned with the picture you have for your future self? This is all about your 'why'. Why does it matter? The answer will probably lie in a sentence that ends with "so that I can…"

Time-bound. This is code for 'this goal has a time limit'. When it comes to time, you don't want the endpoint to be too far away (say, a year) but you don't want it to be a few weeks either. I think a three-month goal is a good compromise, and it's no coincidence that my private programmes run over that length of time.

SMARTER goals are even better because you add 'exciting' and 'rewarded' to the mix.

E is for Exciting. Make sure your goal energises you and is personally motivating. Focus on what will be possible for you when you reach your goal. How will it really feel when you achieve what you set out to do? Get really fired up by your goal.

R is for rewarded. Your goal should have a clear non-food reward for getting the job done. This can be something tangible like a spa day or a gift to yourself or it could be subtler and more intrinsic, like the reflected joy or happiness that comes from mastering a skill, or the satisfaction of a job well done. If there's no real benefit or reward for reaching your goal, your motivation is likely to dip. How will you reward yourself? What will feel like a real win? Remember, since we're in the world of wellness, I'm not talking about having a big blow-out at the end of a diet but something more nourishing of the soul.

Complete the following statements/questions to help you set your goals:

My goal is _____

_____

_____

It is clear and specific in the following way _____

_____

_____

I know if I've achieved it when _____

_____

_____

I can measure success by _____

_____

_____

My goal is realistic because _____

_____

_____

I will have achieved my goal by [__/__/____] _____

_____

_____

What excites/ inspires me about my goal is _____

_____

_____

I will reward myself when I reach my goal by _____

_____

_____

When I achieve my goal, I will feel _____

_____

_____

Finding your why

There are a lot of books designed to help you figure out what your true-life purpose is. This exercise is nowhere near as profound but is still important for anyone who has goals.

I want you to take one of your goals and ask yourself why you want to achieve it. The real 'why' is never in the first few things that spring to mind so, if you think, 'yep, I'll just rush through this little exercise and move onto the next thing', don't waste your time here. You need some time and patience for this one but it's really worthwhile.

The real answer to why you want something might surprise you.

So, the exercise… there's no magic, just sit with the question and write down (yes, another writing task) absolutely everything you can think of about why this matters. Don't settle for any fewer than five or six reasons why your goal is important. I want you to keep going until you have five or six as a minimum. The kind of answer that is your real *why* is the one that is given a bit grudgingly - like, 'okay, it's because I want to ….'

You will never regret taking 20-30 minutes to figure this out. If you have a goal, it will 10X your chance of actually reaching it.

Here's a word of warning: the feeling you *should* do something is not the same as your *why* and the two ought never to be confused. Whatever the opposite of empowering is, you do that every time you 'should' yourself. 'Should' makes you feel told off, naughty or bad about yourself, which is never the right mindset to start any new plan at all. You need to want to do it because you have got clear on what the consequences are of staying put.

Imagine your way to success

You're unlikely to get what you want long term without your destination being a bright and shining beacon that keeps you pressing on even on the darker days.

Visualisation can help.

When you visualise something, over time your subconscious mind will re-programme itself to achieve your goal. There was a famous study with basketball players conducted at the University of Chicago in 1996. First, they worked out what the percentage of 'made' free throws was. That's how many balls went through the hoop. Then they divided the players into three groups. Over the course of 30 days, one group were told to practise taking shots at the hoop for half an hour a day; another group to stay home and do nothing and the third group had to come to the gym, close their eyes and imagine taking successful shots for half an hour. They all then repeated the same test they had done at the beginning.

Those that did nothing did not improve. No surprise there. Those who practised improved by 24%. Practice makes perfect and all that. But those who just imagined they were practising improved by pretty much the same degree (23%). Mind blown. It's a popular technique used by many sports professionals across all kinds of different sports, and it works because the same neurological pathways fire in both instances. Steal this trick yourself by making your goals vivid.

Here's how to do it

This exercise is a bit like imagining your life as a movie so find somewhere quiet to sit and close your eyes if you want to. Revisit your goals and imagine this is your actual reality. Not, 'I want to be' or 'when such and such happens' but like it is your reality. You're actually *there*, experiencing all the good things. You're at your happy weight, you wake up feeling bright and rested after a good night's sleep, you're smiling and happy, the cats come in for a little snuggle to tell you they're ready for breakfast, so you head downstairs to feed them and to make yourself a cuppa. You sit outside on the bench in the garden soaking up the morning sun, knowing you have 15 minutes to enjoy it before the rest of the house starts making demands. Or whatever.

Obviously, your own imaginings might be different. Run your scenario through your mind just like you were watching it on a cinema screen. What do you see? What can you hear? What are people saying? What do you feel? Build up the picture in your head until it is really vivid and you are feeling really good.

This is a powerful technique to reinforce your goals and will supercharge the likelihood of success but you have to practise. I'll show you how to actually do that in an easy way in a moment, but first I need to tell you this:

Motivation is a funny thing and it changes over time

By the time people are spurred into action and ready to part with their money in order to reach their goal (and working with a coach is an investment in your health), the pain of where they are starting is significant enough for them to eat a diet of only kale for two weeks if it came to it. My programmes are never ever punishing and nor do they feature weird foods you hate - just saying. But the point is, most people can do all sorts for a short period of time to move away from the mental or physical pain they are experiencing.

Then things start to change for the better because they've been following their programme. All those things that bothered them before start to improve. Typically, my clients find their energy improves, the hot flushes dial down in frequency (and sometimes vanish altogether), they begin sleeping through the night and the fog starts to lift. They're maybe not where they want to end up, but they're getting there.

Since the pain of where they started has diminished, the desire to move away from where they are is less great - after all, life is pretty good. There's a little more complacency and this is the danger point. There's no longer an urgency to move away from something. Now it becomes critical to focus on where you are heading. That place you are heading is what's in your vision. The more vivid it is, the easier the pull towards it will be.

This is the reason willpower does not work when it comes to reaching your goals. Far sooner than you think, you need to have a strong vision to begin living into so, rather than be repelled by where you started, you are being energetically pulled towards a compelling future. So you really must do that vision work and keep it alive.

The 30-second mindset trick that keeps you motivated

If clients come back to me after a period of time of not working together and their good habits have started to slide, this is what usually has happened and here's how to fix it. Frequently, it's one of these things or both:

1. They've likely forgotten 'what's in it for me?' so are no longer taking committed action.
2. They aren't taking their self-care seriously and, if they are doing any, it is not enough. When this happens, food and wine become something more than food and wine. They become big; a crutch, and you look for these things to be the answer to all kinds of problems.

Here's a really easy trick to help with point one. I must warn you that it's so easy and obvious it feels it cannot possibly be the fix - but it is. Trust me on this. The trick is a daily affirmation and it will take no longer than 30 seconds. Not one of those 'you are worthy of greatness' messages (you are by the way, that's a given, and if you like all of those positive suggestions, go for it).

According to the Merriam-Webster dictionary, the verb 'affirm' means one or all of the following: to validate or confirm, to state positively, to assert (something, such as a judgement or decree) as valid or confirmed, or to show or express a strong belief in or dedication to (something, such as an important idea).

In my world, an affirmation is something you say to yourself every single day to remind yourself 'what's in it for me' to continue on this path. Remember, no one ever does anything without knowing this vital piece of information.

Your daily affirmation is like setting your internal GPS for success every day. It's the thing you need to hear to keep motivated. It is essential in keeping you focused on your goal and yet it's such a tiny demand on your time, so don't skip this.

How to create your affirmation

This is what it looks like in real life: take your inspiration from the vision you created for yourself earlier as well as your goals and attach an action to it.

The formula is this:

What I want + what I must do to get there = success.

You don't want a giant list of goals. Choose the main one. And the action might be something like 'every day I make the best food choices, I take one step closer to my goal'. Put this all into present tense, which means saying it as if it already were the case rather than a hope or wish. Why? The basketball people.

Let's give that a whirl: I am slim and strong and feeling full of energy. I am confident in who I am and I love my life. And every day I make the best food choices ….

Obviously amend to suit whatever you have in mind but make it feel real. I'm just giving you an idea of the appropriate length. Take a little time to work on what you want to say then write it down so you don't forget it.

Research shows the best way to achieve goals like this is to either say them out loud or write them down (if you are the kind of person who loves to journal). Both make your affirmation much more real. The official name for this is the label-feedback mechanism, in which you are more likely to recall something that is spoken out loud than not. Or 'selective attention', in which a goal spoken out loud results in a greater focus on it and increased likelihood of retaining the information. Bottom line: you're more likely to stick to your plan.

When you start to take actions not aligned with your vision, what has happened is that you can no longer remember 'what's in it for me?' If this starts to happen, bring back in your affirmations, like they are a daily business meeting with yourself, and this will help you get back in the zone.

Fake it till you make it

The key to success is to practise, practise, practise rewiring your brain by creating new, positive thoughts. Not there yet? Fake it! Right now you might now be having some doubts about how this is going to make a difference. Perhaps that it's all very well creating something new but it won't work because you don't believe it to be true.

Put yourself in the place where you can see where you want to go, where you need to be, and then act as though you are already there.

Have you heard of laughter yoga? Essentially this is a training in 'voluntary laughter', which differs from 'spontaneous laughter' because you force yourself to laugh until at some point this forced laughter turns into real and contagious laughter. It's a real 'fake it till you make it' situation. The same goes for what we are doing here.

> **10-second recap**
> In order to get what you want, you need to be specific about your goals - otherwise what you have is a vague wish. You need to also figure out why your goals are important to you, really imagine yourself achieving them, and use the power of affirmations (daily reminders) to keep your goals fresh, which keeps you consistently moving forward.

CHAPTER 18
PLANNING & PREP

Now you have your head in the right place, we need to talk about the practicalities of making change possible. If you've tried to make changes to what you eat or your lifestyle before, you'll know that creating the right environment around you helps enormously. Without proper planning and preparation, any goals are just wishes. You need a plan. You'll be used to this kind of approach, of course, because that's how all the regular diet books go about the business of change - create the physical environment by getting rid of any foods you're choosing not to eat from the cupboards and writing yourself a strict meal plan from which you must never deviate.

We'll talk about this soon but, if you skipped the previous chapter on getting your head in the right place first, I recommend you do go back to read it. Sorry to sound all bossy about it but this book is not put together in a specific order by chance. What you believe about yourself and the reason why change is important for you are significant if you want to make changes long term.

There is some solid science behind this rather than anecdotal evidence. The concept is called *Logical Levels of Change* and the theory is based on the work of logician and philosopher Bertrand Russell, later refined by Gregory Bateson and Robert Dilts. (This level of detail might be helpful for the pub quiz, you never know.)

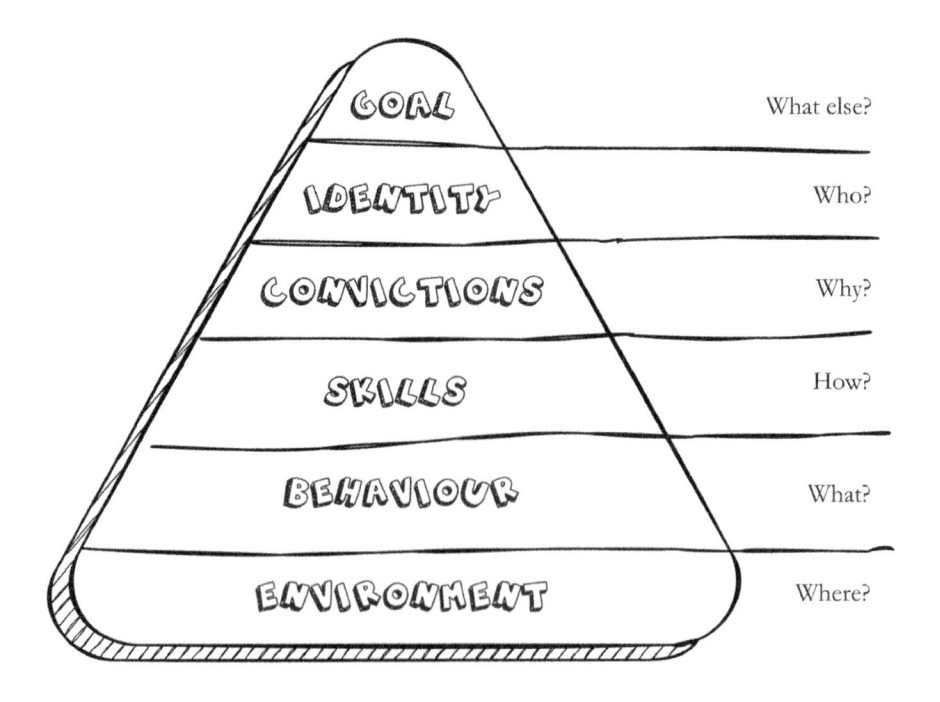

```
      /\
     /GOAL\                What else?
    /------\
   /IDENTITY\              Who?
  /----------\
 /CONVICTIONS \            Why?
/--------------\
/    SKILLS     \          How?
/----------------\
/   BEHAVIOUR     \        What?
/------------------\
/   ENVIRONMENT     \      Where?
----------------------
```

The typical diet approach requires you fix the things nearest the bottom of the pyramid like your environment and your behaviour. It has you change your environment (remove the cakes and biscuits from the kitchen cupboards, join a gym) to help you reach your goals. Your behaviour is what you actually do in the given environment such as tweaks you make to your food intake or the classes you sign up for at the gym. This is where typical diets stop, and this is their downfall. So, in picking up this book, you are already ahead. Plus you are stretching your capabilities by reading this book and acquiring new knowledge that will further inform your actions - you will be able to make the best choices for you based on what you now understand about the way your body works. But back to the 'pyramid of change'.

The rest of the pyramid tackles some of the harder, more philosophical stuff that goes to your very core like 'why does this matter?' (your convictions) and 'who am I?' (your identity).

If you believe yourself to be 'a person who cannot lose weight no matter what you try, guess what will happen? You'll stay stuck. When you can see where you want to be - really see it - it's within reach. We talked about this in the last chapter.

For the purpose of fitting the Logical Levels theory to my narrative, this is the part of the book where we talk about organising your house and your life so that things work in your favour and not against you. You see, you have already done the hard work.

This next part is the easy bit.

Plan, plan, plan

Have you ever embarked on a journey to eat healthier, only to be derailed by an empty fridge, rushed mornings, or the lack of a meal prep for work? Life's unexpected twists can throw off even the best intentions. Without a strategic weekly meal plan, you're leaving it to chance whether your fridge or cupboards will have the right ingredients. And if you don't prioritise your meal times? That protein-packed breakfast or dream lunch can easily slip through the cracks.

The only thing that happens when you don't get a plan in place is chaos reigns and, even if you're a person who thrives on being spontaneous, this is not good for your goals. And it also does not make for harmonious living since you're wide open to the dreaded question 'What's for dinner?' (to which you're forced to say, 'Go forage – if you can find it, you can have it' more often than is normal). Hello downhill spiral and here's a reminder of what that looks like – I've said it before, but it bears repeating:

There's no time for breakfast (or nothing healthy). Toast it is. I had no other options, okay?

Recriminations. What is wrong with me? Can't even get breakfast right. Going to be good from now on.

Mid-morning. Starving face off. Ooh, biscuits.

More recriminations. Shoulda, coulda, woulda had the fruit and nuts. Right, I can get this back, and I'll be better tomorrow.

Is it lunch yet? Cough up £10 in that little sandwich place. Don't have time for stuff with a fork today. Got to eat at my desk so it has to be sandwiches and crisps. This is definitely the last day I do this.

Ooh, it's Sandra coming round with the Devon fudge brought back from her holidays. Tomorrow, I am officially getting back on this. Just one piece, okay, I'll take a second for later. Thank you.

Back home. Why am I so hungry today? Hunts through cupboards. Ugh.

Nothing looks appealing. Not really in the mood for cold chicken breast and a jar of leftover pickles.

Sod it. Today was a total disaster. We'll get a take-away. I'm going to start all over tomorrow. I'll set the alarm so I get up in time for breakfast. I'll make my own lunch tonight. Tomorrow I will be a planning goddess.

Ooh, that thing's on TV. Don't want to miss that. Bed.

This is what happens. This is your life. If not exactly like it, an approximation. I don't say that to be critical. Sometimes it's my life, too. There's nothing wrong, it's just not what you want and it sure as hell won't help you get what you want in your life.

Yes, if you've been paying attention you'll have spotted that you read these exact words back in Chapter 6 but I think a reminder is always good as so much is at stake. The fix is making a weekly food plan of what's going to be on the menu (even if sometimes it's not entirely adhered to). This will reduce dinner-time stress and keep you on track with your goals.

Planning your planning

Here's the thing about planning: you need to actually plan to plan. At the risk of being all Martha Stewart planning your planning is not just something you *could* do if you have 'extra' time in the week. It's a must-do and one that needs its own diary date. It's one of the first things I get my clients to do.

Having worked as an editor in interior magazines for years, I realise that, while Martha Stewart may have been a goddess in my world, you may not know who she is. She was the queen of home entertaining, design and decor, and organisation in the US for decades.

The reason is, it's easy to get thrown off by events, situations, relationships and tasks that insert themselves into your already busy life. So, if you're committed to changing the way you eat, losing weight and, in fact, making any change in your life, download my *Ultimate Guide to Planning* - it's free and you can find it on the Resources page at the back of the book. Print it out. Save a tree by not printing the cover but get the food plan pages in front of you.

Work backwards. If you want to do the shopping on a Monday evening after work every week, when is the *latest* you can sit down to write the plan?

When is the *best* time for you to write the plan? The ideal scenario is you have a regular time for the shop (online delivery or in person trolley dash) and a regular time for the planning so that both become habit and, eventually, you are doing them on autopilot.

In practice, it will help to actually put the time into your diary rather like you would an important work meeting. When can you do that? Get that in the diary now.

What to eat
When it gets to the planning of the plan, look at what's possible. What do you want to eat? What works with all the different commitments your family has this week?

What if you don't have time to do this?
I cannot be clear enough, not having time is a false economy. Not planning will see you waste even more time thinking and on multiple shopping trips so you need to get this fixed as a priority. If you are convinced you don't have time, I want you to humour me and do a little exercise to work out where the time is slipping away. I have worked with a lot of everyone, even business women at the top of their game - CEOs, directors and managers. There's not been a woman yet who genuinely has not had the time for it when we looked deep enough.

How do you actually spend your time?
If you're one of those super-busy people who always finds themselves complaining they don't have time, you're going to need to deal with that. 'Not having time' is a story we tell ourselves or other people in order not to have to take responsibility for – or actually have to do – a particular thing. Sorry to be the one to break it to you, but you make time for what you prioritise in life. Anything else is just an excuse and we both know it. This is said with love, not judgement. I waste an astonishing amount of time when I don't check myself.

If you're reading this thinking, 'Yes, but…' let's take a look at how you are spending your time. Be aware, this really could be life changing.

Ask yourself how you feel about how you are spending your time. Are you in control of your time? If today's pattern continues, will the future you be satisfied?

I'm going to gift you a free book of printable planners. Find it on the Resources page at the back of the book. It's packed with useful pages you can print individually to help you plan and shop your meals. The page I want you to navigate to now is the daily planner.

For the next week, use the daily planner. Log everything. It's enlightening (if a little frightening) to see where your hours actually go. It's quite common for my clients to discover they are spending hours every day scrolling on social media but, because it isn't always a solid batch of time and more a series of 10-minute stretches, the lost minutes - although they are piling up - are unaccounted for. To be clear, there's nothing wrong with scrolling on social media or aimless browsing (not before bed, we cleared that up already) but thinking you have no time then realising hours of it are spent online is something different. It is an awareness and, with awareness, comes choice. Do you want to do that or do you want to do something different?

When you do this exercise, you'll see where you're losing time or being inefficient with it. Face the facts, see where time gets wasted, and feel its impact. (This is designed to be empowering not preachy, so I hope it's coming across the way it's intended.) Are these time-drains ruining your health goals? Are you piling up unnecessary expenses because you're always grabbing breakfast on-the-go?

Realigning your time can free up hours for the healthy habits you think you don't have time for. This planner isn't just pages and dates; it's your blueprint to build the life you want.

The weekly review

I can't recommend highly enough a weekend braindump of all the things that are coming up the following week for you or anyone else in the household so you can see the terrain you're dealing with ahead of time. What are the meetings, sports matches, social events, what's on your exercise schedule, and what about the boring stuff like cleaning and getting the food shop done? Plot it all out on a calendar.

Once you know what's on, you can plan your life much better. You can prep or part-prep meals or lunches ahead of time so you don't have excuses. This will save you a lot of money. You can spot where you can fit a walk in around meetings, for example, to avoid spending the whole day at your desk. I'm sure you get my drift.

> **Don't drown in lack of time - create more of it**
>
> It's easy to get into a spin when things seem very busy. Although the mind is very complex, it is also much more easily fooled than you might think. Let me share a trick I use with a lot of my clients. I'll share Natalie's story because it really was a game changer for her and might help you, too.
>
> Natalie is a conveyancing solicitor who was really struggling to eat well because she was super stressed and very busy. It was the run-up to Christmas and it was during the pandemic times when the UK Government made it very attractive to buy and sell houses thanks to a giant cut in the Stamp Duty tax, and her practice was extraordinarily busy. The busyness was very real, and all her internal talk was about how little time she had. It engulfed her whole life. She was showing up every day as a person who is so busy, and that led to 'I am so busy I can't take my own lunch to work and have to buy whatever I can find in the corner shop'. It affected how she related to her staff because really busy people haven't got time for patience.
>
> My request to her was to catch herself every time she said something to herself about not having time or being busy. Not to berate herself, but to take a second to back-pedal and replace 'I'm so busy' with 'I have all the time in the world'. Even though this was clearly not the case and work *was* frantic, she had a huge shift in the experience of what it was like to be in her life. She felt so much calmer, and she reacted to people and situations in a much more composed fashion because she had

> all the time in the world.
>
> You might doubt this could work. It might seem laughable, even. Take a leap of faith and try it. Note: take care not to make yourself wrong for saying anything negative.
>
> Simply rewind and say to yourself 'I have all the time in the world' – or whatever feels right to you. It is not a test. Just do your very best and I think you will surprise yourself.

Create the right environment

Does your kitchen create the right environment for all this magic to happen? Does your bedroom feel like a relaxing space to be?

When your environment supports your health goals, it makes things significantly easier. I'm not suggesting you need a new kitchen because it's the ageing units or your lack of an air fryer that is lurking behind your weight gain. On a superficial level, having an ordered kitchen where you can easily find what you need is helpful.

Similarly, when the contents of the cupboards are heavy on the kinds of foods you want to minimise, that makes your endeavours a lot harder. If you have a partner and/or children who love snacks, think about where these are stored. Since I don't know your circumstances and everyone is different, I'm just going to make a vague suggestion that all the crisps and biscuits (and other foods of that kind) go in one cupboard and ideally not a cupboard you have to go into all the time because it also contains the tinned tomatoes. If there's a single location the biscuits and crisps live and you choose not to go there, that's easy. If these foods are scattered in every cupboard you have, you'll have reminders pretty much every time you open a door of 'here's what you're missing out on' and it will mess with your head.

Apply the same logic to other environments you need to support your goals. Example: bedroom - tidy, uncluttered, with fresh sheets and soft lighting (remember that bit about dimming the lights) is much more inviting than a cluttered space. If you exercise at home, make the space work for you. If the garage has some gym stuff in it, for example, but you have to climb over the kayak and your kids' sporting equipment to get to the exercise bike or weights, working out will feel much harder work and you'll more easily find a reason for not doing it.

> **10-second recap**
>
> Having a clear vision of what you want matters, and now you need to organise your environment so it supports your goals. That means planning what you will eat and when, even if you occasionally deviate from the plan. You *must* plan your planning so you can be sure you have the food you want to eat in cupboards when you want it.
>
> Planning also makes it significantly more likely you will find and make time to wind down, de-stress, and get to bed earlier.

CHAPTER 19
ACTUALLY DOING THE WORK

If you've read all the way through to this point, I want to say thank you. Really, excellent job. I appreciate, there is a lot to do and one of the things I know from my private clients is the sheer volume of stuff they *could* do is so overwhelming it feels easier to retreat back to the sofa with the TV remote, a good book, or a glass of wine (and maybe all three) and leave all this undone.

Please don't do that. You've come too far.

It doesn't really matter where you start, just that you do.

Where you start and exactly what actions you take will depend on where you are right now. Sorry if that sounds unhelpful. Without meeting you personally, I don't know what your diet looks like, what your stress levels are and so on but let me give you a steer.

Consider starting with sleep - here's why:
Since I'm a nutritionist, you might expect me to say do the food work first. You can absolutely start fixing any of the pillars in this book: food, sleep, stress management, exercise. The reason I am suggesting maybe look to sleep first is that, when you are well rested, all kinds of previously-unimaginable things start looking like they might be possible.

Prioritising your sleep means you'll wake up feeling more refreshed and motivated. You'll have the headspace to take on new things and you'll be more resilient, which makes all of the other pillars easier to do as time goes by. If you make getting to bed earlier your new thing, chances are you will then also have a headspace for planning and prepping what you are going to eat, so that makes the food piece of the puzzle easier.

Because sleep is pivotal to weight management, too, consider that if you're not getting seven hours plus sleep on a regular basis, you're not getting the most from any weight loss efforts.

Knowing what I know, that would be my best advice to you. But also knowing what I would be like in your position, I would likely want to start changing my diet because it seems the most logical.

Then move onto the food stuff

Now you know what you know about food and your midlife metabolism from our earlier chapters, where seems the best place to start? I advise starting with fixing what goes on at breakfast. When you reliably start the day with a protein-rich breakfast, you are less likely to experience cravings later in the day.

You can then work through the different meals and tackle the work that needs to be done. I know I've repeatedly said ideally you want three meals a day and no snacks but if you really need a snack, what I really *don't* want is for you to go off and eat the things marketeers want you to think are healthy. Need some snack inspo? I wrote something just for you and you can find it in the Resources section at the end of the book.

Planning will be key

If you don't actually make the time for planning and shopping, good luck. It might seem unnecessarily dogmatic but unless you have a plan, it will be sheer luck or a fair wind that helps you make changes stick. In any book you care to read on creating habits, creating a path with no friction works. That's code for 'if it feels hard, you won't do it.' Since you learned all about this in the last chapter, I shan't labour the point but planning helps you create a great framework for the magic to happen.

So, sleep, good planning, and eating well. From there, you can branch into whatever makes the most sense next. If you know you're under stress or have been in the last handful of years, go there. Otherwise, work out how you can get strength training into your life.

I frequently find this strategy works for many people for a handful of weeks. You're starting fresh, everything feels do-able, you're enthusiastic and desperate to move forwards. Within the first few weeks, you *must* do the work about why this matters because no one ever does anything without knowing 'what's in it for me?' (WIIFM).

WIIFM is a big deal in marketing and anyone trying to sell you anything will be following a framework that sells you on the benefits to you personally of buying this or that. WIIFM is not just a list of features a product might have, it is the actual benefit of having the actual thing in your actual life. So, as far as a new food and lifestyle programme goes, WIIFM is not that you are going to focus on or reduce certain foods or have a specific amount of sleep or take up strength training, the answer lies in what follows after the words 'so that I can…'

Consider, you are 'selling' these changes to yourself on a daily basis so you need to work out why this matters. And you will also need to remind yourself daily because otherwise the chance of your going back to 'business as usual' and doing whatever you were doing before that didn't work is too great.

You absolutely *must* do the affirmations

Even if you think this is woo woo. One of the biggest things women face in trying to lose weight or change their diet in order to fix something about their health is consistency. That means doing something for long enough to get the effect you want even if (and especially when) you are not sure if things are changing. Trust the process. Seek personalised help, if you need it (check out the Resources at the end of this book for contacts) but keep going. The scale is not the only measure. There are much better ways to monitor progress. This brings me neatly onto…

Focus on the non-scale victories

Given you are reading this book in the first place, you'll know those tricks you used to roll out to shift a few pounds a decade or so ago no longer work. It *is* possible to lose weight in midlife, but the rules are different and maybe also they are more complicated. Because weight is connected not only to how many calories you eat but *what* you eat, *when* you eat, and *what else* is going on in your body: blood glucose levels for starters, your basal metabolic rate, how much sleep you've had, how stressed you are, whether you've done a poo (seriously, that can make the difference of a couple of pounds), and other variables, just going by the scales is going to be no fun. Instead, think about the little wins beyond the scale - like more energy, sleeping better, fewer headaches, less brain fog, fewer hot flushes, beloved clothes fitting you again, and so on.

Create your own scale

To see how you're doing in different areas of your life, I like to use a wellness journal and score how I'm feeling about different aspects of my life on a weekly basis or even sometimes how successfully I feel I'm adhering to different habits I want to track like mindfulness, exercise, and so on. You can use a journal use it to track the severity of symptoms, too, if you like.

Try a scale of 1 to 6, with a score of 1 meaning it's not a noticeable problem and 6 being the symptom is as bad as you can remember. Measure up to three of the most obvious symptoms, and throw in a 'general wellbeing' score, too, which measures how it feels to be you.

Even when weight loss takes longer to show on the scale (because often the last thing on the tree is the fruit), you can see how well the rest of your life is shaping up. Although you might be concerned about your weight, feeling clear headed, more springy, and more *you* is always a joy.

Don't wait until someday to start loving your life. There is only now

Fixing your midlife metabolism is about making changes to the way you eat, sleep, rest and move, and starting to feel great from the inside out. But how about giving yourself a confidence boost and learning to feel great from the outside in?

In midlife, it becomes a bit of a vicious circle. Women often don't like or even recognise the person they see staring back at them in the mirror so they stop treating her to the good things, like nice smellies, new clothes, and so on. My personal and professional view is focussing on feeling and looking good for yourself *right now* is essential. It's very much something you can be in control of, and it needn't be expensive. Stop waiting to take better care of yourself in that fictitious 'someday'.

Start with a deep cleanse of your wardrobe, which I suspect might be harbouring all kinds of clothing you don't even like yourself in. Marie Kondo – author of *The Life Changing Magic of Tidying* – is a genius and I lean heavily on her for inspiration in this area. A wardrobe cleanse that starts with tops, bottoms, hung-up items like dresses and jumpsuits, jackets and such like, then moves through underwear, handbags, accessories and shoes, is the first place she advises her clients to go when they embark on sorting out their homes (and their lives). She describes it as a "rite of passage to a new life" and she's right.

Use your "intuitive sense of attraction" (Marie Kondo again) to work your way through your clothes and begin to discard anything you haven't worn for a year or more, that doesn't feel great on you or that feels dated (jeans, for example, have a sell-by date as styles seem to last only for a few years - if you don't believe me, watch an older film and you'll soon agree), clothes that are worn-out or damaged and can't be fixed. Trust your judgement here. If a garment does not feel right, something must be wrong with it: the colour, cut, style or pattern. Check your shoes aren't dated or tired and that they match your outfits.

Wearing the right colours for your skin tone makes a huge difference to how you look and how good you feel in something. Chances are you've been complimented recently on an article of clothing that you hadn't considered was all that. It was probably that the colour looks so good on you. As a side note, the colours that suit you really can change over the years as skin colour alters a little as you lose the youthful glow and maybe you've even changed your hair colour.

It might be you have some big gaps in your wardrobe contents yet you don't want to go out and buy new stuff. What I would say is this: don't wait until you reach your target weight to buy anything new. If you're trying to lose weight, just buy one outfit that you look good in and that makes you feel great. Consider sites like eBay and Vinted for bargain, good-as-new items.

Giving yourself permission to look good – whatever that means for you – is a significant statement. Taking care of yourself is like telling yourself 'I really matter'. And you do. When you start loving yourself properly again and treating yourself well, it's the gateway to a whole other kingdom.

An endnote

So that's it from me, my midlife friend. I hope I can call you that since we've now spent so long together. I wish you all the very best in creating the health and the life you want. I'm always here for you: follow me on socials at @foodfabulousnutrition, read the blog at foodfabulous.co.uk, join a group programme or treat yourself to a midlife metabolism makeover and work with me one-to-one.

Now is a good time to stop and summarise this whole midlife metabolism business in just a few lines:

The rules of weight loss change from perimenopause onwards. It's no longer about calories but about how much you eat, what you eat, how you eat, when you eat, reducing stress, sleeping well, and building muscle. To get all of these changes into your life, you need to start with why this matters to you, you need to remind yourself regularly so you can do the work consistently enough to see the changes you want, and you need to see this as an amazing opportunity to create a life you truly love.

I know that it can feel overwhelming trying to keep yourself feeling well. The amount of advice online is massive and it's hard to know who is qualified to dispense it, and whether they have any vested interests. Nutrition and lifestyle medicine - an approach you have been learning about in this book - is the answer to pretty much everything. It won't replace conventional medicine but, when it comes to midlife and menopause, you cannot just take a pill, pop on a patch or rub in some gel. I know that might be the last thing you want to hear right now but the good news is that you really can do something to improve pretty much every marker that goes a bit haywire as you get older by making some reasonably simple adjustments to what you eat and how you live. No one is asking you to fall in love with kale or eat knitted yoghurt.

Your body is an amazing piece of kit and all the symptoms you might be experiencing are your body talking to you. It's up to you to listen.

REFERENCES

Chapter 1 How does your metabolism get broken?
Baker C (2022) Research briefing: obesity statistics, House of Commons Library, accessed:
https://commonslibrary.parliament.uk/research-briefings/sn03336/#:~:text=Obesity%20is%20usually%20defined%20as,%2C%2059.0%25%20of%20women) Accessed: 19th July 2023.
Number of people living with diabetes in the UK tops 5 million for the first time (2023) Diabetes UK.
https://www.diabetes.org.uk/about_us/news/number-people-living-diabetes-uk-tops-5-million-first-time. Accessed: 19th July 2023.
Diabetes and Women (2022) Centers for Disease Control and Prevention. https://www.cdc.gov/diabetes/library/features/diabetes-and-women.html#:~:text=Diabetes%20increases%20the%20risk%20of,%2C%20kidney%20disease%2C%20and%20depression. Accessed: 19th July 2023.
Deaths registered summary statistics, England and Wales (2022, Office for National Statistics. https://www.ons.gov.uk/peoplepopulationandcommunity/birthsdeathsandmarriages/deaths/articles/deathregistrationsummarystatisticsenglandandwales/2022#:~:text=For%20females%2C%20dementia%20and%20Alzheimer%27s,the%20exception%20of%20COVID%2D19. Accessed: 19th July 2023.
Yusuf A et al. (2004) Effect of potentially modifiable risk factors associated with myocardial infarction in 52 countries (the INTERHEART study): case-control study, *The Lancet*, Sep;364(9438):937-52, doi: 10.1016/S0140-6736(04)17018-9.

Chapter 2 Get back in control of your blood glucose

Alemany M (2021) Estrogens and the regulation of glucose metabolism, *World Journal of Diabetes*, Oct 15; 12(10): 1622–1654, doi: 10.4239/wjd.v12.i10.1622.

Berlanga-Acosta J *et al.* (2020) Insulin resistance at the crossroad of Alzheimer disease pathology: A review, *Frontiers in Endocrinology* (Lausanne) 2020;11:560375. https://www.ncbi.nlm.nih.gov/pmc/articles/PMC7674493/. Accessed: 21st July 2023.

Ma LH, Lin GZ, Wang M. (2017) Association between estrogen and female patients with Alzheimer's disease: a meta-analysis, *International Journal of Clinical and Experimental Medicine*, 10: 135-141.

Litwak SA, Wilson JL, Chen W, Garcia-Rudaz C, Khaksari M, Cowley MA, Enriori PJ (2014) Estradiol prevents fat accumulation and overcomes leptin resistance in female high-fat diet mice, *Endocrinology*, 155:4447–4460.

Chapter 3 How weight loss works

Kong LC *et al.* (2013) Insulin resistance and inflammation predict kinetic body weight changes in response to dietary weight loss and maintenance in overweight and obese subjects using a Bayesian network approach, *American Journal of Clinical Nutrition*, Dec 98(6):1385-94.

Chapter 4 Your metabolism, calories & hunger

Richard Feinman and Eugene Fine (2004) A calorie is a calorie violates the second law of thermodynamics, *Nutritional Journal*, doi.org/10.1186/1475-2891-3-9.

Kekwick A, Pawan GL (1956) Calorie intake in relation to body-weight changes in the obese, *The Lancet*, Jul 28;271(6935):155-61. doi: 10.1016/s0140-6736(56)91691-9.

Fung J (2016) *The Obesity Code*, London, Scribe Publications, p29-47.

Suminthran P (2011) Long-term persistence of hormonal adaptations to weight loss.
New England Journal of Medicine, Oct 27;365(17):1597-604.

Lee I, Djoussé L, Sesso HD, Wang L, Buring JE (2010) Physical activity and weight gain prevention, *JAMA*, March 24; 303(12):1173-9.

Hagobian TA, Sharoff CG, Stephens BR, *et al* (2009) Effects of exercise on energy-regulating hormones and appetite in men and women, *The American Journal of Physiology - Regulatory, Integrative and Comparative Physiology*, Feb;296(2):R233-42.

Chapter 5 Other metabolism wreckers

Marizzoni M *et al.* (2020) Short-chain fatty acids and lipopolysaccharide as mediators between gut dysbiosis and amyloid pathology in Alzheimer's disease, *Journal of Alzheimer's Disease*, 2020; 78 (2): 683, doi: 10.3233/JAD-200306.

Turnbaugh PJ, Ley RE, Mahowald MA, Magrini V, Mardis ER, Gordon JI (2006) An obesity-associated gut microbiome with increased capacity for energy harvest,
Nature, Dec 21;444(7122):1027-31, doi: 10.1038/nature05414.

Ferolla SM, Armiliato GN, Couto CA, Ferrari TC (2014) The role of intestinal bacteria overgrowth in obesity-related nonalcoholic fatty liver disease, *Nutrients*, 2014;6(12):5583-5599, doi:10.3390/nu6125583.

Hasani A, Ebrahimzadeh S, Hemmati F, Khabbaz A, Hasani A, Gholizadeh P (2021) The role of Akkermansia muciniphila in obesity, diabetes and atherosclerosis, *Journal of Medical Microbiology*, Oct;70(10), doi: 10.1099/jmm.0.00143.

Al-Obaide M *et al.* (2017), Gut microbiota-dependent trimethylamine-n-oxide and serum biomarkers in patients with T2DM and advanced CKD, *Journal of Clinical Medicine*, Sep 19;6(9):86, doi: 10.3390/jcm6090086.

Wilders-Truschnig M *et al.* (2008), IgG antibodies against food antigens are correlated with inflammation and intima media thickness in obese juveniles, *Experimental and Clinical Endocrinology & Diabetes*, 116(4):241-5.

Chapter 8 Foods that help you lose weight

Acosta L, Byham-Gray L, Kurzer M, Samavat H (2022) Hepatotoxicity with high-dose green tea extract: effect of catechol-o-methyltransferase and uridine 5'-diphospho-glucuronosyltransferase 1A4 Genotypes, *Journal of Dietary Supplements*, doi:10.1080/19390211.2022.2128501.

Lopez-Garcia E, van Dam RM, Li TY, Rodriguez-Artalejo F, Hu FB (2008) The relationship of coffee consumption with mortality, *Annals of Internal Medicine*, 148, 904-914, doi: 10.7326/0003-4819-148-12-200806170-00001 .

Koot P, Deurenberg P (1995) Comparison of changes in energy expenditure and body temperatures after caffeine consumption, *Annals of Nutrition and Metabolism*, 39 (3): 135–142, doi: 10.1159/000177854.

Bracco B, Ferrarra JM, Arnaud ML, Jéquier E, Schutz Y (1995) Effects of caffeine on energy metabolism, heart rate, and methylxanthine metabolism in lean and obese women, *American Journal of Physiology*, Oct;269(4 Pt 1):E671-8.

Acheson KJ et al. (2004) Metabolic effects of caffeine in humans: lipid oxidation or futile cycling? *American Journal of Clinical Nutrition*, Jan;79(1):40-6. doi: 10.1093/ajcn/79.1.40.

Costill DL, Dalsky GP, Fink WJ (1978) Effects of caffeine ingestion on metabolism and exercise performance, *Medicine & Science in Sports & Exercise,* 10(3):155-8.

Ochoa-Rosales C *et al.* (2023) C-reactive protein partially mediates the inverse association between coffee consumption and risk of type 2 diabetes: the UK Biobank and the Rotterdam study cohorts, *Clinical Nutrition*, doi: 10.1016/j.clnu.2023.02.024.

Gupta JS, Puri S, Misra A, Gulati S, Mani K (2017) Effect of oral cinnamon intervention on metabolic profile and body composition of Asian Indians with metabolic syndrome: a randomized double -blind control trial, *Lipids in Health and Disease*, Jun 12;16(1):113, doi: 10.1186/s12944-017-0504-8.

Shen, J *et al.* (2012) Beneficial effects of cinnamon on the metabolic syndrome, inflammation, and pain, and mechanisms underlying these effects – a review, *Journal of Traditional and Complementary Medicine*, (2: 1) 2012, 27-32, doi: 10.1016/s2225-4110(16)30067-0

Mousavi SM et al. (2020) Cinnamon supplementation positively affects obesity: a systematic review and dose-response meta-analysis of randomized controlled trials, *Clinical Nutrition,* Jan;39(1):123-133, doi: 10.1016/j.clnu.2019.02.017.

McDonald D *et al.* (2018) American gut: an open platform for citizen science microbiome research, *American Society for Microbiology,* 416 198,434, doi: 10.1128/msystems.00031-18.

Chapter 11 Sleep, the game changer

Sundelin T, Lekander M, Sorjonen K, Axelsson J (2017) Negative effects of restricted sleep on facial appearance and social appeal, *Royal Society Open Science*, 4:160918, doi:10.1098/rsos.160918.

Pacheco A, Singh A (2023) Alcohol and sleep, *Sleep Foundation*. https://www.sleepfoundation.org/nutrition/alcohol-and-sleep. Accessed: 30th July 2023.

Sutherland S (2013) Bright screens could delay sleep, *Scientific American*. https://www.scientificamerican.com/article/bright-screens-could-delay-bedtime/#:~:te xt=If%20you%20have%20trouble%20sleeping,to%20blame%2C%20new%20resear ch%20suggests.&text=If%20you%20delay%20that%20signal,says%2C%20you%20 could%20delay%20sleep. Accessed: 2nd August 2023.

Newsom R, Singh A (2023) How blue light affects sleep, *Sleep Foundation*. https://www.sleepfoundation.org/bedroom-environment/blue-light. Accessed: 20th October 2023.

Lucas A, Wilson N (2019) Does television kill your sex life? Microeconometric evidence from 80 countries, National Bureau of Economic Research. https://www.nber.org/system/files/working_papers/w24882/w24882.pdf. Accessed: 23rd October 2023.

Manchester Evening News (2013) TV's a bedroom turn-off. *Manchester Evening News*. https://www.manchestereveningnews.co.uk/news/greater-manchester-news/tvs-a-be droom-turn-off-1016884. Accessed: 20th October 2023.

Chapter 12 How to sleep better

Scheer FAJL, Hilton MF, Mantzoros CD, Shea SA (2009) Adverse metabolic and cardiovascular consequences of circadian misalignment, *PNS*, doi:10.1073/pnas.0808180106

St-Onge MP, Mikic A, Pietrolungo CE (2016) Effects of diet on sleep quality. *Advanced Nutrition*, Sep 15;7(5):938-49, doi: 10.3945/an.116.012336.

Paddock C (2013) Caffeine can disrupt sleep hours later, *Medical News Today*, https://www.medicalnewstoday.com/articles/268851#Caffeine-6-hours-before-bed-re duced-sleep-by-at-least-1-hour. Accessed: 30th July 2023.

Ebrahim IO, Shapiro CM, Williams AJ, Fenwick PB (2013*)* Alcohol and sleep I: effects on normal sleep, *Alcohol: Clinical & Experimental Research,* 37: 4, doi: 10.1111/acer.12006.

Thakkar MM, Sharma R, Sahota P (2015) Alcohol disrupts sleep homeostasis, *Alcohol*, 49(4) 299-310, doi: 10.1016/j.alcohol.2014.07.019.

Fairbrother K, Cartner B, Alley JR, Curry CD, Dickinson DL, Morris DM, Collier SR (2014) Effects of exercise timing on sleep architecture and nocturnal blood pressure in prehypertensives, *Vascular Health and Risk Management*, Dec 12;10:691-8. doi: 10.2147/VHRM.S73688.

Dolezal BA, Neufeld EV, Boland DM, Martin JL, Cooper CB (2017) Interrelationship between sleep and exercise: a systematic review. *Advances in Preventive Medicine,* 2017:1364387. doi: 10.1155/2017/1364387.

Gradisar M, Lack L, Wright H, Harris J, Brooks (2006) Do chronic primary insomniacs have impaired heat loss when attempting sleep? *The American Journal of Physiology - Regulatory, Integrative and Comparative Physiology,* Apr;290(4):R1115-21. doi: 10.1152/ajpregu.00266.2005.

Healthline (2019) Having trouble sleeping? Try a hot bath before bed, *Healthline.* https://www.healthline.com/health-news/having-trouble-sleeping-try-a-hot-bath-befor e-bed. Accessed: 30th July 2023.

Chapter 13 - Stress & your metabolism

Nicolle L, Woodriff Beirne (2010) The healthcare futurescape: how did we get here and where are we going? In: Nicolle L, Woodriff Beirne A, eds. *Biochemical imbalances in disease.* London, Singing Dragon, p38-51.

Wudarczyk OA, Earp BD, Guastella A, Savulescu J (2013) Could intranasal oxytocin be used to enhance relationships? Research imperatives, clinical policy, and ethical considerations, *Current Opinions in Psychiatry*, Sep;26(5):474-484, doi: 10.1097/YCO.0b013e3283642e10.

Scheele D, et al. (2012) Oxytocin modulates social distance between males and females, *The Journal of Neuroscience,* 32 (46) 16074-16079; doi:10.1523/JNEUROSCI.2755-12.2012.

Chapter 14 Create an anti-stress action plan
Sung MK, Lee US, Ha NH, Koh E, Yang HJ (2020) A potential association of meditation with menopausal symptoms and blood chemistry in healthy women: a pilot cross-sectional study, *Medicine* (Baltimore), Sep 4;99(36):e22048. doi: 10.1097/MD.0000000000022048.

Chapter 15 The right exercise
Fung J (2016) *The Obesity Code*, London, Scribe Publications, p48-56.
Hagobian TA, Sharoff CG, Stephens BR, et al (2009): Effects of exercise on energy-regulating hormones and appetite in men and women. Am J Physiol Regul Integr Comp Physiol. 2009 Feb;296(2):R233-42.
Minnis DPT (2023) How Much Muscle Mass Should I Have, and How Do I Measure It?, *Healthline*, https://www.healthline.com/health/muscle-mass-percentage#calculations. Accessed: 23rd October 2023.
Berin E, Hammar M, Lindblom H, Lindh-Åstrand L, Rubér M, Spetz Holm AC (2019) Resistance training for hot flushes in postmenopausal women: a randomised controlled trial, *Maturitas,* Aug;126:55-60. doi: 10.1016/j.maturitas.2019.05.005.

Chapter 16 - Getting a bit more active
Yamamoto, N., Miyazaki, H., Shimada, M. *et al.* (2018) Daily step count and all-cause mortality in a sample of Japanese elderly people: a cohort study, *BMC Public Health,* 18, 540, doi:10.1186/s12889-018-5434-5.

Chapter 17 - Get your head in the game
Lupyan G (2012) Linguistically modulated perception and cognition: the label-feedback hypothesis, *Frontiers in Psychology*, 2012; 3: 54. doi: 10.3389/fpsyg.2012.00054.

RESOURCES

You're still here ☺ That's good.

At various points in this book I talked about some brilliant stuff you might find helpful on your journey to fixing your midlife metabolism. Firstly, although this is not a recipe book, I do want to give you the option to check out some delicious **low carb recipes** based on the concepts I talk about in the book. You'll find a bunch of them over here on the resources page of my website . You can also use your phone camera and hover over the QR code below, then hit the button to be spirited off to the website.

From this page, you'll also be able to download the ***Ultimate Guide to Menu Planning*** completely free. You can also skip straight to the download page here: https://www.foodfabulous.co.uk/planning-guide. Plus links to anything I mention below. (I say this because, at any time, the links to other people's websites could change but mine won't).

In Chapter 2 (Get back in control of your blood glucose), I told you about various ways of monitoring your blood sugar levels. You can buy a blood glucose monitor in pharmacies and online retailers.

If you like the idea of using a **continuous glucose monitor**, I recommend Lingo and Veri. Both offer great apps that help you make sense of the squiggly graphs the machine will chuck out.

ABOUT THE AUTHOR

Ailsa Hichens is a UK-based Registered Nutritional Therapy Practitioner and Health coach specialising in menopause and midlife health. She has over 10 years' experience helping women improve their health and happiness. She is passionate about health education and regularly delivers webinars and talks to companies and in the community. Her approach is evidence-based and practical, and her goal is to help 'normal' people put the science of feeling great into their daily lives.

She is always researching, keeping her knowledge up to date and sharing practical applications of the science on her website and social media channels.

Website: https://www.foodfabulous.co.uk
Instagram: https://www.instagram.com/foodfabulousnutrition/
Facebook: https://www.facebook.com/foodfabulousnutrition/
Newsletter: https://www.foodfabulous.co.uk/food-fabulous-vip-list

Printed in Dunstable, United Kingdom